I0439271

Diabetes Diet

Diabetes Management Options Includes a Diabetes Diet Plan with Diabetic Meals and Natural Diabetes Food, Herbs and Supplements for Total Diabetes Control Delicious Recipes Covering Breakfast, Lunch, Dinner and Snacks

By John McArthur

Copyright

ISBN-13:978-1495900815

ISBN-10:1495900819

Natural Health Magazine

www.naturalhealthmagazine.net

The information in this book is provided for educational and information purposes only. It is not intended to be used as medical advice or as a substitute for treatment by a doctor or healthcare provider.

The information and opinions contained in this publication are believed to be accurate based on the information available to the author. However, the contents have not been evaluated by the U.S. Food and Drug Administration and are not intended to diagnose, treat, cure or prevent disease.

The author and publisher are not responsible for the use, effectiveness or safety of any procedure or treatment mentioned in this book. The publisher is not responsible for errors and omissions.

Warning

All treatment of any medical condition (without exception) must always be done under supervision of a qualified medical professional. The fact that a substance is "natural" does not necessarily mean that it has no side effects or interaction with other medications.

Medical professionals are qualified and experienced to give advice on side effects and interactions of all types of medication.

Table of Contents

Copyright..2

Foreword...11

Do We Have A Death Wish? 12

Types of Diabetes 15

   Type I and II Diabetes 15

   Three Other Types of Diabetes.. 17

Diagnosis – Signs and Symptoms...18

Causes of Diabetes 22

   Causative Factors in Type 1 Diabetes (IDDM) 22

   Causative Factors in Type II Diabetes (NIDDM)........................ 24

Complications of Diabetes 27

   Hypoglycemia 27

   Diabetic Ketoacidosis... 28

   Hyperosmolar coma 28

   Non-Ketogenic Hyperosmolar Syndrome............................... 29

   Glycosylated Proteins and Diabetic Complications 29

   Sorbitol and Diabetic Complications 30

   Atherosclerosis 30

Diabetic Neuropathy...31

Diabetic Retinopathy 32

Diabetic Nephropathy (Kidney Disease)...............................32

Diabetic Foot Ulcers...33

Conventional Medical Treatment.....................................34

Natural Treatment Options..37

The Diabetes Diet Treatment 37

Beneficial and Harmful Foods...39

The Benefits and Importance of Dietary Fiber 41

Diabetes and the Glycemic Index 42

Hidden Sugars 44

Say No to Refined Foods 44

The Diabetes Nutritional Supplement Treatment...................45

Chromium Picolinate...46

Vitamin E 46

Vitamin C...47

Vitamin B6...48

Vitamin B12...48

Magnesium 49

Silymarin..50

Niacin and Niacinimide 50

Biotinide 50

Potassium 51

Manganese 52

Zinc 52

Essential Fatty Acids.. 52

Alpha-Lipoic Acid.. 53

Carnitine 53

Vanadium 53

Coenzyme Q10 54

Amino Acids 54

Digestive Enzymes.. 54

The Diabetes Herb Treatment 54

Bitter Melon 55

Onion (Allium Cepa) and Garlic (Allium Sativum)................ 55

Salt Bush.. 56

Gymnema Sylvestre 57

Bilberry.. 57

Huereque 58

Stevia.. 58

Fenugreek Seeds 59

Ginkgo Biloba 59

Additional Treatments for Diabetes 60

Exercise 60

Remember This: 63

Exercise Precautions 63

Chelation therapy 65

Oxygen Therapy 65

Traditional Chinese Medicine 66

Ayurvedic Medicine 68

20 Recipes for Breakfast, Lunch Dinner and Snacks 70

5 Breakfast Options to Start Your Day 71

Turkey Sausage and Scrambled Eggs on a muffin 71

Oatmeal with Berries, Apples and Pecans 73

Low Fat Bran Muffins 75

Ham Cheese and Broccoli Dish 77

Oatmeal Waffles 80

Healthy Breakfast Shake 82

5 Easy Lunch Meals 83

Chutney Chicken Wrap 83

Grilled Lamb Burgers..85

Chicken and Almond Salad with Rye Bread 87

Roast Beef Sandwich..89

Turkey and Potato Salad 91

5 Quick and Easy Meals for Dinner................................93

Baked Garlic Chicken with Butter Beans.........................93

Traditional Spaghetti and Meatballs............................95

Cashew Vegetable Stir Fry 97

Lamb Stew with a Middle Eastern Twist...........................98

Shrimp Vegetable and Creamy Garlic Pasta 100

5 Healthy Snacks for Anytime....................................102

Homemade Granola Bars..102

Delicious Cookies – Without the Sugar...........................104

Chewy Brownies..106

Peanut Clusters 108

Pumpkin and Raisin Bars..110

Fats: The Good, the Bad and the Ugly.....................112

Good Fats and Bad Fats 112

The Good Fats..113

Monounsaturated Fats 113

Polyunsaturated Fats 113

The Bad and the Ugly Fats 113

Saturated Fats 114

Trans Fats 114

Omega Fatty Acids 115

What are Omega Fatty Acids? 115

Getting More Essential Fatty Acids in Your Diet 119

The Diabetic's Shopping List...120

Don't Buy this 120

Glycemic Index 122

Breakfast Cereal... 122

Staples.. 123

Bread.. 124

Snacks & Sweet Foods 125

Legumes (Beans).. 126

Vegetables 127

Fruits 128

Dairy... 129

Bibliography 130

More Books by John McArthur...131

Foreword

Research has shown that diabetics can control their condition very effectively with the right diet, natural supplements and herbs. They can live a normal and healthy life as long as they adhere to certain measures.

A low-fat, high-fiber, whole-food diet packed with vegetables, fruits, nuts, seeds and lean protein is encouraged.

Diabetic foods should ideally be low GI (Glycemic Index) foods rich in key nutrients such as calcium, magnesium, vitamin A, vitamin C.

The advice in this book will give you a comprehensive understanding of diabetes as well as information on conventional and natural treatment options.

Included in the book are 20 recipes to help you prepare delicious meals and snacks.

Being a diabetic does not mean that your diet needs should be monotonous – filled with bland and unimaginative food. You will see that there are many ways to prepare healthy and delicious meals.

Do We Have A Death Wish?

If you are not suffering from diabetes yourself, chances are that you know someone who struggles with some form of the disease. Statistics show that the incidence of diabetes is on the rise. This dramatic and disturbing increase can largely be attributed to how our diet has changed in modern society. Fast food has become more popular and it has become increasingly more acceptable to include large amounts of processed food and sugar in our diet.

You will find that most people who struggle with this condition have been struggling to make healthy diet and lifestyle choices over a very long period of time. This condition does not suddenly appear overnight. Diabetes is more prevalent in the Western world, but as the Western-Style diet spreads to other places, so does the incidence and rise of Diabetes. Chris Kilham is a Medicine hunter who researches medical remedies all over the world. His words on the global struggle with diabetes are thought provoking:

A virtual diabetes pandemic is sweeping the world, with record levels of obesity and diabetes crippling the health of hundreds of millions of people globally. As horrible as this is, what is even worse is the sobering evidence that most people appear unwilling to take the lifestyle steps that can prevent this killer disease. Do we have a death wish?

The Diabetes foundation recently released statistics regarding this condition in the US:

- Approximately 26 million Americans have Diabetes.

- It is estimated that 79 million people have pre-diabetes.

- Diabetes is responsible for a quarter of a million deaths in the United States each year.

- Medical costs for diabetes amount to more than $218 Billion Annually.

This proves that Diabetes is indeed a serious problem. The question we are now faced with is two-fold. What lifestyle changes can we make and maintain to avoid contracting this condition? If a diagnosis has already been made, what can be done to ensure a long and healthy life? As we become aware of the facts surrounding diabetes and what can be done in terms of treatment, it becomes clear that in most cases there is much hope.

In the information that follows, I hope to shed light on this condition and on the challenges that those who have it are faced with. I will also discuss many options surrounding possible treatments, both conventional and therapeutic.

Types of Diabetes

There are two major types of Diabetes namely Type I and Type II. There are several similarities between the two but in essence they are very different. The common thread running through both of them is that they are characterized by abnormal levels of sugar and glucose in the blood. Being properly informed will help you put a treatment strategy in place that will enable you to manage the specific condition that you have.

Type I and II Diabetes

Type I Diabetes is an auto-immune disease known as Insulin Dependent Diabetes Mellitus (IDDM). IDDM is also called Juvenile-onset diabetes as it occurs mainly in children and adolescents. It is less prevalent than Type II Diabetes as it accounts for only 10 percent of all cases. There is uncertainty as to what triggers the initial onset of IDDM. It is however generally believed to be caused by destruction or injury to the insulin-producing beta-cells. Beta cells are groups of cells that are located in the pancreas. IDDM occurs when these cells are attacked and destroyed by the body's own immune system. A defect in tissue regeneration capacity is also thought to contribute to its onset. Type I Diabetics need to regularly monitor and test their blood sugar levels, which they can control by injecting insulin several times a day. Together with the insulin shots, they need to watch their diet and exercise regularly to avoid the risk of complications.

Type II Diabetes, also known as Non-Insulin-Dependent Diabetes Mellitus (NIDDM), affects as much as 90 percent of people with the disease. These people have a very high insulin level, which indicates a loss of sensitivity to insulin by the cells of the body. Although genetics play a role, there are several other factors which may trigger the onset of Type II Diabetes. Some of these include:

- Being overweight.
- Lack of exercise.
- High Blood Pressure.
- Poor Diet.

Obesity is a huge risk factor. An Australian Scientist by the name of Kelly West, M.D., PH.D said: "The cause of type II Diabetes is usually obesity; the preventative, and often the cure, is leanness." As many as 90 percent of people with NIDDM struggle with obesity. Although this is alarming, all hope is not lost. The great news is that normal healthy blood sugar levels can be restored gradually as the person makes deliberate lifestyle changes to achieve his/her ideal body weight. The correct diet can control type II Diabetes, and even though many doctors still resort to using drugs and insulin, it is still the best method of treatment.

Three Other Types of Diabetes

There are three other types of diabetes. The first, Secondary Diabetes, is a form of diabetes that results from other conditions such as hormone disturbances, drug use, pancreatic disease, and malnutrition. As it is not the main condition, it should improve when the primary problem is dealt with.

The second, Gestational Diabetes, is quite a common health problem amongst pregnant women. During pregnancy, cells are less responsive to insulin because of hormonal changes. Therefore, the pancreas needs to work harder at producing sufficient insulin. If it is unable to deliver, the result is that the mother's blood glucose levels rise too high and she ends up developing gestational diabetes. A woman struggling with gestational diabetes can take comfort in the fact that it should go away once her baby is born.

The third type, Impaired Glucose Tolerance, is commonly referred to as pre-diabetes. The reason for this is that people with this condition have blood glucose levels that are higher than what they should be but lower than those of a person with full blown diabetes. These people are not considered diabetics as such, but they are at risk of becoming type II diabetics if they do not make prompt diet and lifestyle changes.

Diagnosis – Signs and Symptoms

Let's take a look at the most common signs and symptoms that accompany Diabetes. Type I and II exhibit very similar symptoms. The difference is that with Type I symptoms may develop very quickly, leading the patient to investigate and treat their specific condition before there are too many complications. Type II can lurk about in the patient's body for a few years before there are enough noticeable symptoms to lead them to make the discovery and ultimately seek treatment.

It is very important that Type I Diabetics are made aware of their condition as soon as possible. Because this is an autoimmune disease that attacks beta cell within the pancreas, the patient will eventually stop producing insulin. The result of this is that symptoms develop very quickly and they then face the life-threatening risk of falling into a diabetic coma. With Type II Diabetes the hormone insulin is still being produced. The problem is that the body is not able to effectively make use of the insulin that is available. Because there is still a small amount for the body to utilize, symptoms take much longer to develop.

Type I and II Diabetes have the following symptoms in common:

- Increased Thirst: If you have this symptom it could be an indication of a different problem. However, because this is one of the earliest symptoms of diabetes it is better to get it checked out early on.

- Hunger: People who have developed diabetes will notice an increase in appetite. They will also begin to notice weight loss. Eating more and losing weight at the same time should be a cause for concern.

- Frequent Urination: Because diabetes causes increased thirst, you will drink more fluids which will lead to more frequent urination. Frequent urination could also be attributed to other conditions so be on the lookout for other signs of diabetes if you suspect it. A diabetics' urine is sweet –smelling due to elevated sugar levels.

- Fatigue and lethargy: Because our lifestyles have become so busy, we easily overlook fatigue and blame the urge to drag ourselves around on other things. Remember that fatigue should never be persistent. If you are struggling with constant fatigue you should definitely investigate. It is one of the telltale signs of diabetes.

- Blurred Vision: This symptom is a result of high blood glucose levels which cause damage to some of the small blood vessels within the eye.

- Heavy, labored breathing: Although respiratory problems are usually responsible for this symptom, it is also a symptom of diabetes.
- Stupor and unconsciousness: Diabetes that has been left to get out of control for a very long time could lead to this.

If you have been struggling with some of the above mentioned symptoms and your doctor decides to do a more thorough investigation, there are several steps that will be taken to make a diagnosis. Usually your doctor will do different tests to determine what your blood glucose levels are. You will be required to do an overnight fast so that your fasting blood glucose level can be tested the next day. If it is below a certain point on two separate occasions, you will be diagnosed with diabetes.

There are two specific tests that might be done. The most common test is called the Glucose Tolerance Test (GTT). If this is your doctor's test of choice you will be required to ingest 150 grams of carbohydrates every day for three days prior to the day of testing. The night before, you will need to do an overnight fast. Your blood glucose levels will then be measured the next day. The results will determine whether or not you have diabetes.

There is an even more sensitive test known as the Glucose-Insulin Tolerance Test (G – ITT). This test is more expensive but is often preferred, as just determining blood sugar levels is not always sufficient in diagnosing a blood sugar disorder. The GITT measures both blood glucose levels as well as insulin levels. If there is a problem with the way your body metabolizes sugar, this test will certainly pick it up.

If after undergoing the above mentioned tests you are diagnosed with some form of Diabetes, it is not the end of your life. It simply means that you will need to make some important and perhaps drastic lifestyle changes to make sure your condition doesn't worsen. It is always tough to make behavioral changes but if you persevere it will become easier to make the right choices over time. Your body will certainly appreciate healthy meals, some level of exercise, less processed fatty food, and sufficient rest. Diabetes is controllable most of the time so the power to make a difference in your health and to turn things around will be in your hands.

Causes of Diabetes

Diabetes causes vary greatly as there are many factors that may influence whether you contract this illness or not. Things such as genetics, family history, ethnicity, lifestyle, and environmental factors all play a role. Each form of Diabetes has its own set of possible causes. Let's take a more detailed look at those causes and how they may induce different forms of diabetes.

Causative Factors in Type 1 Diabetes (IDDM)

Although diet and lifestyle are usually the main factors in the development of NIDDM, genetics also play quite a significant role in select cases. Certain people are more susceptible to contracting diabetes because of their genetic makeup. They often have a hereditary predisposition to the destruction or injury of their insulin producing beta cells together with the inability by their pancreas to generate new beta cells. Injury to these cells is usually a result of viral infections, autoimmune reactions, and/or free radicals.

There is quite strong evidence to support the theory that viral infections may lead to the development of IDDM later on. This was suspected because people seemed to be diagnosed with diabetes around the same time that viral infections were going around. Viral Infections like congenital rubella, mumps, hepatitis, etc. are more prevalent from October to March. Beta-cells within the pancreas can be infected and destroyed by viruses, which could also induce antibody attack.

The greatest causative factor in IDDM is autoimmune reactions. The process of autoimmunity is when your body develops antibodies against the beta cells within your pancreas. As many as seventy-five percent of all IDDM sufferers have this problem. The development of antibodies is most likely a reaction to cell destruction as a result of viral infections or other illnesses. Each person has a different degree of autoimmune reactions as well as differing capabilities within their bodies to repair the damage to beta cells.

Some studies have shown that exposure to cow's milk in infancy has the ability to bring on Type1 Diabetes by triggering the autoimmune response. Tests have been done on animals to try and prove that this is not the case, however tests done on humans have produced conflicting results. Studies show that people with Type I Diabetes were most likely breast-fed for less than three months and were usually exposed to cow's milk and solids before four months. The protein found in cow's milk can be ingested by breast fed babies. It is therefore advisable for breastfeeding mother's to avoid cow's milk if they have a history of diabetes in their family.

Causative Factors in Type II Diabetes (NIDDM)

NIDDM sufferers have one primary problem and that is that they have developed insulin insensitivity. Several factors including genetics, obesity, viral infections, food allergies, stress and diet all contribute to the loss of insulin sensitivity. There is enough insulin in the bloodstream of a NIDDM patient but the insulin cannot do what it is supposed to do because of beta cells that have become unresponsive.

Most people with NIDDM are obese. There has been a remarkable rise in the incidence of diabetes in parallel with obesity. Insulin resistance develops as the patient gains weight, especially around the upper body through bad diet choices, inactivity etc; up to 85 percent of people diagnosed with NIDDM are overweight or obese. A medical professional at Ulm University, Dr. Ernest Pfeiffer, made this statement: "It's almost a law that any person 30 percent overweight for 30 years will become a diabetic." The majority of NIDDM patients can drastically improve their situation as they actively work to decrease their body fat percentage. This will either completely cure them or at least restore some level of insulin sensitivity. It is interesting to note that diabetes develops not as a result of how much food was eaten, but rather the quality of the food. Processed foods that are high in calories and basically devoid of fiber and essential nutrients contribute greatly to the gradual development of insulin insensitivity and ultimately NIDDM. There are two stories that I am going to share with you that shed light on the extent of the influence that diet has on the development of NIDDM.

There is a small Island on the Pacific known as Nauru. The island's inhabitants lived a very simple life for the longest time with a diet that consisted mainly of fruits such as bananas and yams. During this time diabetes was virtually unheard of in Nauru. A few years ago Phosphate was discovered on the Island. This brought great wealth to the people of the Island, who then went on to completely change the way they lived their lives. Part of this change included a drastic change in their diet. They replaced a diet that usually consisted of fruits and vegetables with a diet very high in carbohydrates, sugar, and fat. Over time, the incidence of Type II Diabetes started to rise dramatically. A study was done by the World Health Organization that shows that as much as 50 percent of the population between the ages of 30 and 64 now has diabetes.

Another story that illustrates the influence that diet has in the development of NIDDM happened in England during World

War II. There was a time when a food shortages forced people to have to cut out sugar, flour, excessive meat protein and fats. During that time there was a 50 percent drop in the amount of people who died from diabetes. These stories only go to prove that in the majority of cases, diabetes is caused by diet as opposed to genetics.

Studies have been done that show a connection between fetal health as a result of the mother's diet and the incidence of NIDDM and IDDM. Murray and Pizzorno explain:

Recent population based evidence supports the concept that the nutritional status of the mother during pregnancy plays a role in determining whether the child will develop both types of diabetes later in life.

Mothers who consume too many calories during their pregnancy put their unborn child at risk of getting some form of diabetes later on. The data from different studies show that when a pregnant mother's blood glucose levels are controlled and monitored, the chances of their child contracting diabetes is greatly reduced. The data collected shows an almost 50 percent drop in the incidence of diabetes in mothers who maintained normal health blood sugar levels throughout their pregnancy.

Complications of Diabetes

There are many complications that could arise from diabetes. Both acute and chronic complications usually arise when a patient has been unwilling or unable to effectively keep blood sugar levels under control. There is a significant drop in the incidence of complications in those who have been able to do so. Murray and Pizzorno explain: "...monitoring and controlling the degree of elevations in blood sugar (hyperglycemia) is critical to the prevention of the major diabetic complications. This goal cannot be stressed too much."

It is important for diabetics to be aware of the extent and type of complications they could face if blood sugar levels are not adequately controlled. This will help them to remain vigilant and to avoid becoming negligent over time in treating their condition. I will elaborate on the most common acute and chronic complications faced by diabetics.

Hypoglycemia

Hypoglycemia is more common in type I diabetics because of the insulin therapy they need to be on. It is usually triggered by too much insulin, skipping meals, or over-exertion. It is crucial that the amount and type of insulin being administered is monitored properly to lower the risk of hypoglycemia. There are different symptoms for daytime and nighttime episodes of hypoglycemia. These are the symptoms that diabetics need to be on the lookout for during the day: hunger, excessive sweating, shaking, and a feeling of uneasiness. Nighttime symptoms include bad dreams, night sweats, and/or headaches.

Diabetic Ketoacidosis

Diabetic Ketoacidosis is more common in type I diabetics. When NIDDM patients do not have sufficient insulin in their bloodstream to break down glucose, which the body needs for energy, fat is broken down instead. As the fats are broken down, there is a gradual buildup of ketones which are a byproduct of fat breakdown. Ketones are toxic and will eventually cause high levels of acidity in the body. This can lead to a coma and other metabolic issues. There will be symptoms leading up to the coma or other more serious side effects. These symptoms include extreme thirst, unusual tiredness, nausea, vomiting, and increased urination. If diabetics suspect Ketoacidosis they can do a simple urine test at home to measure the amount of ketones in their urine.

Hyperosmolar coma

This is a very serious complication that is not to be taken lightly. 50% percent of hyperosmolar coma cases result in death.

This coma is brought on by severe dehydration as a result of insufficient fluids, over-exertion, infection, or surgery

Non-Ketogenic Hyperosmolar Syndrome

This complication has a 50% mortality rate and is considered a very serious medical emergency. Certain events or situations lead to a diabetic patient becoming severely dehydrated. The causes vary greatly and can range from pneumonia, a stroke, burns, certain drugs, insufficient fluids etc. This syndrome usually develops slowly over a few weeks or days and exhibits symptoms such as thirst, frequent urination, and signs of dehydration. The dehydration signs to be on the lookout for are dry mucous membranes, loss of elasticity in the skin, low blood pressure and increased heart rate.

Glycosylated Proteins and Diabetic Complications

The process of binding glucose to proteins is called glycosylation. Glycosylation changes the make-up of some of the body's proteins as well as their function. The glycosylation that takes place in diabetics affects the proteins in their red blood cells, lenses, and the myelin sheath that insulates and covers nerve cells. Too much glycosylation disrupts cell functions, inhibits molecule binding, and inactivates enzymes.

Sorbitol and Diabetic Complications

When glucose is metabolized by the body sorbitol is produced. This process occurs in everyone but in diabetics it is accelerated. Sorbitol is fine in moderation but as soon as it becomes excessive it starts to wreak havoc on the nerves, kidneys, and eyes of diabetics. As it builds up it gradually depletes the body's supply of vitamins, minerals, and amino acids. Too much sorbitol also attracts water into the body's cells. This is what ultimately leads to nerve damage, vision problems, blood vessel damage, and kidney problems.

Atherosclerosis

Atherosclerosis is the hardening of arteries that occurs when fat, cholesterol and other unwanted substances build up on the walls of arteries and form hard structures called plaques. Over a period of time these plaques could block arteries and start causing symptoms throughout the whole body. This condition is usually something that develops with age, but can happen in younger patients as a result of other illnesses like diabetes. Diabetics stand a chance of dying from this condition - one that is three times greater than your average person. If you are a diabetic it is important for you and your doctor to have game plan in place to reduce the risk of a heart attack or stroke. One of the best things any diabetic can do to reduce the risk is to gradually reduce cholesterol levels. This can be done by:

- Minimizing the amount of animal products being consumed. This will automatically cut out harmful saturated fats and cholesterol.
- Making sure that there is an increase in the consumption of fiber-rich plant foods such as grains and vegetables.
- Reducing overall body weight with a healthy diet and regular exercise.
- Making overall lifestyle changes like giving up smoking and cutting down on coffee, both caffeinated and decaffeinated.

A few positive changes can make all the difference in ensuring a diabetic lives a long and healthy life.

Diabetic Neuropathy

Diabetic neuropathy is quite a common complication of diabetes that damages the nerves in the body that allow you to feel pain. This nerve damage occurs when blood sugar levels have been high for a long time. It can be quite painful but most people experience mild symptoms.

Diabetic neuropathy most often damages nerves in the legs and feet of diabetics. Symptoms of nerve damage typically

31

include pain and numbness in the extremities and complications with the digestive tract, urinary tract, heart, and blood vessels. Once again the risk of having to deal with this complication can be greatly reduced by controlling blood sugar levels and living a healthy lifestyle in general.

Diabetic Retinopathy

Diabetes that is left to get out of control results in high levels of blood sugar. This is called hyperglycemia. When this blood sugar accumulates in a diabetic's blood vessels, the blood flow to their organs is either damaged or hampered in some way. When the blood flow to their eyes is affected they might develop diabetic retinopathy that could lead to blindness. When the flow of oxygen to the eyes is hampered the body tries to compensate by forming new fragile blood vessels in the retina. Sometimes these vessels are damaged which results in bleeding into the eye. To stop the bleeding diabetics can go for laser treatment. Unfortunately the treatment often destroys much of the retina, which is crucial for sight. Diabetic retinopathy is one of the leading causes of blindness in the USA. One in 15 type II diabetics and one in 20 type I diabetics will develop retinopathy.

Diabetic Nephropathy (Kidney Disease)

Diabetes sometimes leads to a patient developing Diabetic nephropathy, which is damage to the kidneys. This happens to be the main cause of death in diabetics around the world. Once again uncontrolled blood sugar levels can lead to blood vessel damage within the kidney. This affects the kidney's ability to function since the vessels that are supposed to filter waste from the body are destroyed. Often times the kidneys will completely stop working leading to kidney failure. For some reason not all diabetics get kidney failure but it is quite common. If care is taken in monitoring a diabetic's blood sugar levels as well as kidney function, the risk of developing this complication will be greatly reduced.

Diabetic Foot Ulcers

Diabetic foot ulcers form when the small blood vessels leading to the foot get clogged. This results in a lack of oxygen which can lead to the development of gangrene and ultimately amputation if treatment isn't prompt. Nerve damage often causes numbness is the feet of diabetics. Because of this it is advised that they never walk around without shoes as cuts and bruises might easily go unnoticed. Diabetics need to make sure that their feet are always kept warm, clean and dry to reduce the risk of foot ulcers.

Conventional Medical Treatment

Conventional medical treatment varies for Type I and II diabetics. Since people with Type I diabetes have an insulin deficiency they require insulin on a regular basis. They need to be injected once or twice daily since insulin taken orally is not absorbed by the body. This treatment for NIDDM has been administered to patients since 1922.

There are currently two different types of insulin therapy available. The first, conventional insulin therapy is done by injecting crystalline insulin once or twice daily, depending on the patient. The type and amount of insulin the patient will need to inject will be determined by several factors including how much food they eat, when they eat, and what their level of daily physical activity is. Although this method is effective the best insulin therapy available is called intensified insulin therapy. This is a more aggressive treatment approach used to keep blood sugar levels under control that should slow down or even prevent the complications that usually come with having diabetes for many years. Patients, who receive this treatment, need to constantly keep track of their blood sugar levels and will be required to inject insulin three to five times daily. The other option they have is to wear an insulin pump. The pump injects a steady supply of soluble insulin into the body all day long through a needle inserted into the abdomen. Fifteen minutes before a meal the patient will need to press the pump manually to inject a larger amount all at once. Although this method is the most effective in mimicking insulin levels that are usually produced by a healthy pancreas there are few minor drawbacks:

- The pump needs to be worn all day which might be an inconvenience at times.
- Patients using this method will need to be very dedicated to carefully monitoring their blood sugar levels at all times.
- Patients will be at a higher risk for hypoglycemia.

The two above mentioned treatments available are always necessary to treat Type I diabetics. People with type II Diabetes have other options available to them. As discussed earlier, most Type II diabetics are overweight or obese. Unlike Type I diabetics, they have no insulin shortage. In fact, their bodies actually secrete four times the amount of insulin usually secreted by the pancreas of a healthy person. The reason for this is that their beta cells have become unresponsive to insulin over time. The excess insulin secreted is their body's attempt to overcome that problem. Since Type II diabetics have developed insulin insensitivity their treatment plan needs to involve steps that will gradually increase their body's sensitivity to insulin. The first treatment option should always be diet therapy. If this is successful, no additional drugs will be necessary. If not, there are drugs available to assist in treatment. These drugs are called oral hypoglycemic agents. Their role is to both stimulate the secretion of more insulin and to increase the body's sensitivity to insulin in general. Unfortunately, these drugs are only effective in about 60 percent of cases. Of those people fortunate enough to see results, only 20 to 30 percent will continue to benefit from the drugs long term as they usually become less effective over time. Another downside to these drugs is that they have quite a few unwanted side-effects, the worst being hypoglycemia. Other side effects include indigestion, nausea, vomiting, headaches, allergic skin reactions, tiredness, and damage to the liver. Because this medication is high risk it should never be used in patients dealing with infections, pregnancy, long term corticosteroid use, injury, or surgery.

Natural Treatment Options

The treatment options available to diabetic patients are abundant and very promising to those who are willing to make the tough decision and changes needed to start the healing process. In this chapter we will look at the many therapeutic treatment options available to diabetic patients. Type I diabetics in particular need to always be carefully monitored and need to make sure they are always on the lookout for symptoms that could point to any complications. Home glucose monitoring and the drawing of blood are necessary to keep track of how they are doing and to decide whether their drug dosages need to be altered. Diabetics who make use of some of the therapeutic treatments that I am going to discuss should be able to adjust their drug dosage as their blood sugar levels start normalizing. With both type I and II diabetes the goal of any treatment approach is to stabilize blood sugar levels. This is easier to accomplish when diabetics actively take control of improving and monitoring their own condition.

The Diabetes Diet Treatment

In our modern society countless people have fallen into the deadly trap of letting their sugar and calorie intake get completely out of control. Diets packed with unhealthy fats are becoming the norm for most people regardless of their age. The number of overweight and obese children is on the rise as well as the incidence of type II diabetes, which used to be more common in older people. It is safe to say that your average American consumes food which will certainly increase his/her insulin resistance over time. The only way this problem can be reversed is if we start becoming brutally honest about how bad diet choices are affecting and possibly shortening our lives.

Your typical American consumes approximately 140 pounds of sugar annually – this is an exorbitant amount of sugar for anyone's body to have to process. Some people's systems are more capable of doing so but others are not as lucky. Every time we eat a bowl of ice cream or drink a can of soda our pancreas works hard to secrete large amounts of insulin into our bloodstream. The insulin's job is to then transport that sugar, in the form of glucose, to our liver, muscle and fat tissue cells for storage. Six percent of people are not able to handle such large amounts of sugar over a long period of time and the result is that their insulin receptors will eventually go on strike and refuse to do their job. The result of that is that excess sugar gets stranded in the bloodstream, resulting in type II Diabetes. The consequences of having this form of Diabetes range from mild to life-threatening as arteries and veins are gradually damaged. Millions of people around the world have contracted type II diabetes so the incidence of kidney disease, eye problems, and nerve damage has also risen significantly. 50 percent of amputations performed in the USA each year are performed on diabetic patients.

More often than not the type II diabetic's ticket to the restoration of a healthy normal life lies in lifestyle changes. Diet and exercise can completely cure or at least dramatically improve type II diabetes. Although this treatment option applies mostly to NIDDM sufferers, Type I diabetics will also see a level of improvement when they make quality lifestyle changes.

Beneficial and Harmful Foods

Two doctors by the name of Dr. Wright and Dr. James Anderson have done extensive studies in their attempt to discover which foods are beneficial and which are harmful to diabetics. According to Dr. Wright:

A diet emphasizing foods high in complex carbohydrates and fiber, such as whole grains, legumes, and vegetables, reduces the need for insulin by slowing and controlling the release of glucose into the bloodstream

Dr. Wright strongly recommends that diabetics stay away from simple carbohydrates such a fruit juices, as well as foods containing refined sugar (biscuits, cakes, pastries etc ;) since these foods cause a rapid and significant rise in insulin levels. This insulin spike in the bloodstream puts unwanted strain on the pancreas. Instead, diabetics should try to include more whole foods in their diet like vegetables, fruits, beans, nuts, grains, seeds etc; these foods are full of nutrients and fiber which all help to lower blood sugar levels. Dr. Wright recommends that diabetics make a point of eating one of every food color each day, for example green peas, orange carrots, red tomatoes, brown rice etc. His reason behind this recommendation:

"If you make sure to eat a nutritional spectrum of colorful foods every day, and if you concentrate on getting those colors from whole foods, you will begin to control high blood sugar with diet."

Dr. Wright also strongly recommends that all diabetics get tested for food intolerances. Some patients could unknowingly be eating foods that are causing autoimmune destruction and inflammation within their bodies. Foods that diabetics have often been intolerant to include chocolate, dairy, wheat, and corn.

Dr. Anderson from the University of Kentucky found that patients who are taking medication to lower their blood sugar level and those who need less than 40 units of insulin are great candidates to control their diabetes by simply eating a diet high in complex carbohydrates and fiber. Your average American consumes only 11-23 grams of fiber daily. Diabetics hoping to see results will need to triple this amount and ensure they drink more water to help increased gas production. When this eating plan is followed the result will be a significant decrease of fats in the bloodstream which will in turn lower the risk of cardiovascular diseases. Dr. Anderson suggests type II diabetics attempt a diet that looks like this:

- 55% to 60% of the daily calorie intake to be derived from carbohydrates (two thirds of these complex carbohydrates).
- 14%to 20% from protein (minimum 45 g daily).
- 20% to 25% or less from fat (10% or less from saturated fat), with only 200 mg or less of cholesterol daily.
- 40-50 g total dietary fiber daily (10-15 g of this as soluble fiber).

The Benefits and Importance of Dietary Fiber

Extensive studies done on the relationship between an unhealthy diet and the occurrence of diabetes clearly shows how closely diabetes and an inadequate dietary fiber intake are linked. One of the most important dietary changes a diabetic needs to make is to significantly increase fiber intake.

Soluble fiber keeps things moving through your gastrointestinal system and is necessary to ensure digestion and nutrient absorption is slowed down. This will cause your body to slowly release glucose from carbohydrates in the body as opposed to the glucose spike that occurs after a low-fiber meal. It is also instrumental in ridding the body of unnecessary bile acids which would have been converted into blood cholesterol.

If you are a diabetic who is attempting to lose weight, fiber will go a long way in helping you do so since it increases the feeling of satiety. Good sources of fiber include most vegetables, oats, nuts, seeds, apples, pears, and beans. The aim should be to consume at least 50 grams of fiber daily. Diabetic who succeeds in doing this should see an overall improvement in their condition in a few weeks.

Diabetes and the Glycemic Index

The notion that only pure sugar causes insulin levels to spike is erroneous. There are many seemingly harmless forms of sugar that have the same effect as pure sugar. A few years ago researchers from the University of Toronto did an evaluation of many different foods to discover what their insulin impact is. They put a rating system together called the Glycemic Index, which helps measure the impact of each and every food on blood sugar levels. Foods with a high rating cause a greater insulin response than those with a lower rating.

The medical director of the Overlook Centre for Weight Management, Dr. R Podell, explains that a diet full of low Glycemic Index foods will certainly be instrumental in keeping insulin lows and blood sugar levels stable. He came to the following three conclusions:

- Foods with a higher rating, causing a higher insulin response, include white bread, bagels, English muffins, packaged flaked cereals, instant hot cereals, low-fat frozen desserts, raisins and other dried fruits, whole milk and whole-milk cheeses, hot dogs, and luncheon meats.

- Foods with a low rating, not causing a high insulin spike, include most fresh vegetables, leafy greens, pitted fruits and melons, coarse 100% whole-grain breads and minimally processed whole-grain cereals, sweet potatoes and yams, skim milk, buttermilk, poultry, lean cuts of beef, pork, and veal, shellfish, white-fleshed fish, most legumes, and most nuts.

- Cooked foods rank higher on the index than raw foods. Similarly, fruits and vegetables that have been juiced or pureed are higher on the index than when eaten whole.

Note:

- A high GI value is 70 or more.
- A medium GI value is 56-69.

- A low GI value is less than 55.

See the last chapter for a detailed list of GI foods and values.

Hidden Sugars

Food manufacturers are generally very careful about including the word "sugar" on the packaging of their sugary foods since this would have a negative impact on sales. Instead, they make use of a few chemical synonyms that mean the same thing – sugar. It is good for diabetics to become familiar with these terms to aid them in making healthy food choices. The most popular synonyms are: dextrose, corn sweetener, fructose, glucose, dextrin, sucrose, high-fructose corn syrup, maltose, maltodextrin, lactose, modified cornstarch, maltose, malt, mannitol, sorbitol, xylitol, sorghum, and fruit juice concentrates.

Say No to Refined Foods

Few things are as satisfying as a slice of white break or a bag of chips, both which contain white flour. Unfortunately these are part of a list of foods that are highly refined and always increase the level of glucose in the bloodstream. Dr. Jonathan Wright, M.D., suggests that diabetics put the following dietary boundaries in place:

- Avoid eating any refined sugar.
- Never eat "junk food."

- Be sure to include protein snacks in your diet between meals.
- Pack your diet with complex carbohydrates.
- Reduce the amount of alcohol, caffeine, and tobacco you take in.
- Make an effort to exercise regularly and lose weight.

The Diabetes Nutritional Supplement Treatment

As the incidence of diabetes has risen over the last few years, people have started looking to alternative therapies. Nutritional supplements are highly beneficial to diabetics and have proven to help lower blood sugar levels and to decrease the risk of complications. The nutritional supplements that that I will be discussing are all useful when taken in conjunction with a controlled and healthy diet. In the treatment of diabetes diet should always be the central focus. Nutritional supplements serve to provide the extra nutrients needed by diabetics. Patients who have chosen this path of treatment have seen some great results. It is certainly worth every diabetic's while to be informed about the nutritional supplement that have proven to improve insulin function and glucose tolerance. Following is a list of some of the great supplements that are recommended:

Chromium Picolinate

This is a great supplement for diabetics to take as it helps stabilize blood sugar levels and improve insulin function over time. In the past, patients who have taken up to 1000mcg daily have seen noteworthy improvements in their condition. Interestingly enough a lack of chromium in non-diabetics results in diabetic symptoms. It only makes sense that this supplement would improve a diabetic's overall condition.

Vitamin E

Vitamin E supplements help to significantly reduce the incidence of complications in diabetics since it has an anticlotting and anti-inflammatory effect and is a powerful antioxidant. Complications such as coronary heart disease, cataracts and kidney problems are often seen in people who have had diabetes for a long time. Vitamin E can delay or prevent these problems as it helps lower blood fats, improve glucose tolerance, and reduces glycosylation.

Some great natural sources of vitamin E are avocados, nuts and seeds, broccoli, wheatgerm oil, and wholemeal cereals. Eating fresh raw foods and taking supplements is the best way to ensure a sufficient intake of Vitamin E.

Vitamin C

Insulin is instrumental in transporting Vitamin C into the cells of our body. When there is a vitamin C deficiency, complications can arise. Since diabetics naturally struggle with insulin function, they usually have a Vitamin C deficiency, even when their diets are packed with great Vitamin C sources. This deficiency manifests itself in vascular disease, bleeding tendencies, a weakened immune system, poor wound healing, and the degeneration of insulin producing cells in the pancreas.

The RDA for Vitamin C in non-diabetics is approximately 60mg. The general consensus is that those with diabetes should try and take between 120 to 250 mg daily if they are going to see an improvement in their condition and a reduced risk of complications. Diabetics who take this much Vitamin C daily will be able to better maintain their eye health by preventing cataracts and might even reduce the amount of insulin they need over a period of time. Most importantly, their immune systems will be strengthened and their bodies will be better equipped to fight infection. Fruits and vegetables like citrus fruit, mangoes, any green sprouting vegetables, green peppers, guavas, potatoes and berries are great sources of Vitamin C.

Diabetics planning on taking a Vitamin C supplement should first go and get their kidney function tested. This is crucial since too much Vitamin C could prove to be toxic to diabetics who are battling renal insufficiency.

Vitamin B6

You may have heard people refer to the B vitamins as immune boosters. This is because this group of vitamins plays a primary role in the production of antibodies, which are required to fight infection – something which diabetics often struggle with. Not only do these vitamins help diabetics fight infection, but they have also been proven to offer protection against neuropathy. Diabetics who are struggling with any form of peripheral nerve abnormalities should certainly be taking a Vitamin B6 supplement. Vitamin B6 has also been shown to offer significant protection against complications such as coronary heart disease and diabetic retinopathy

Diabetics can benefit greatly from Vitamin B6 supplements. According to Dr. Sarah Brewer "All the B group vitamins are beneficial for people with diabetes as they are involved in the processes which produce energy within body cells." Sources of Vitamin B6 include liver meat, oily fish, bananas, nuts, wholegrains, avocados, egg yolk and green leafy vegetables.

Vitamin B12

Vitamin B12 plays a key role in lowering homocysteine levels. Homocysteine is a naturally occurring amino acid found in blood plasma which can cause complications when its levels within the body are raised. Diabetic retinopathy is one of these complications. Doctors have been treating diabetic retinopathy with Vitamin B12 since the 1950's and the results have been astounding. Diabetics can take up to 2mg a day if necessary. No side effects have been reported, even with such a high dosage.

This vitamin is also helpful in the treatment of diabetic neuropathy and can be found naturally in kidney, meat, sardines, dairy products, eggs, and liver.

Magnesium

Magnesium is an important supplement used by the body in the process of glucose metabolism. Most diabetics have a magnesium deficiency and should consider taking a supplement since it could help prevent both retinopathy and heart disease. Diabetics need up to double the RDA of non-diabetics. This amounts to approximately 600 mg a day.

Magnesium helps maintain a healthy cardiovascular system by decreasing the amount of cholesterol and fat in the blood. It is also helpful in preventing retinopathy and atherosclerosis.

Silymarin

Silymarin is a powerful antioxidant found in the herb milk thistle. Studies show that it can help type 2 diabetics by lowering their glucose levels. It also acts as an anti-inflammatory when necessary and has been shown to prevent liver damage and help maintain healthy liver function.

Niacin and Niacinimide

According to Dr. Wright "Niacinamide, one of the B vitamins, is the number one nutrient for treating Type 1 Diabetes." Several experiments done on animals suggest that niacinamide may actually slow down or completely stop the development of Type 1 Diabetes. This is because niacinamide helps slow down the demise of beta cells and plays an important role in glucose tolerance. This naturally reduces the extent of blood vessel and organ damage caused by raised blood sugar levels.

Biotinide

Biotin is part of the B group of vitamins and is used by the body to synthesize and metabolize fatty acids, amino acids, stress hormones, genetic material and glucose. When taken as a supplement by diabetics, Biotin serves to improve insulin sensitivity and most importantly enhance the activity of glucokinase, which is an enzyme used by the liver to process glucose. Studies show that type 1 and 2 diabetics who took this nutrient enjoyed lower blood sugar levels and improved glucose control. Over time some were even able to adjust their insulin requirements.

The recommended dosage of biotin for diabetics is anything between 0.15 mcg and 1mg. Food sources include egg yolks, wholegrains, fish, liver, cauliflower, meat and nuts.

Potassium

All diabetics should be eating a diet that is full of potassium as it is helpful in improving insulin sensitivity, secretion and responsiveness. The incidence of heart disease, atherosclerosis and cancer is reduced in patients who receive a lot of potassium, either through supplementation or diet.

It is preferable for diabetics to receive potassium through their diet as potassium salts can have unpleasant side effects like vomiting, nausea, diarrhea and ulcers. Although most diabetics can handle a lot of potassium, those with kidney failure will not be able to process large amounts and might suffer the consequences of potassium toxicity.

Potassium is found naturally in fresh fruit, seafood, vegetable juices, mushrooms, potatoes, peppers, spinach, lima beans and peas.

Manganese

We all need manganese as it is involved in thyroid hormone function, blood sugar control, and energy metabolism. Diabetics naturally only have half of the manganese found in healthy individuals so they need to be taking manganese supplements. The recommended dosage is 30 mg a day.

Zinc

Zinc has proven to be useful in improving insulin function and in reducing the risk of certain diabetes related complications. Since it plays a crucial role in the storage, synthesis, and secretion of insulin, a deficiency will certainly affect insulin function within the body.

Food sources containing zinc include seafood, offal, wholegrains, eggs, cheese, seafood and brewer's yeast.

Essential Fatty Acids

Both omega-3 and omega-6 have proven to benefit diabetics. Omega-3 helps type 2 diabetics by enhancing insulin secretion and preventing the hardening of arteries. It also reduces vascular complications and insulin resistance. Gamma-linolenic is an omega-6 fatty acid that has proven to help prevent diabetic neuropathy.

Omega-3oils can be found in pumpkin seeds, soybeans, flaxseed oil, beans, spinach, winter squash, broccoli, cauliflower, as well as mackerel, salmon and cod fish oils. The primary omega-6 oil is called linoleic acid and can be found in peanuts, sesame, corn, safflower, wheatgerm, cotton seed, vegetable and sunflower oils.

Alpha-Lipoic Acid

Alpha-Lipoic acid has successfully been used by doctors to treat adult-onset diabetes for more than 30 years. It is not effective when taken orally so needs to be administered intravenously. A dose of 1,000mg should help to lower insulin resistance and improve the cells ability to use glucose by as much as 55 percent.

Carnitine

There is evidence that Carnitine could play a role in slowing down or even preventing diabetic ketoacidosis. Diabetics who have taken Carnitine supplements also noticed an increase in HDL-cholesterol levels and a decrease in total serum lipid levels.

Vanadium

Vanadium can be found in dill seed, grains, unsaturated vegetable oils and black pepper. Since it mimics insulin, it may improve the diabetics' condition by helping regulate blood sugar.

The recommended daily dosage is between 5-2 mg daily. The supplement form to look out for is called Vanadyl Sulfate.

Coenzyme Q10

All human cells contain coenzyme 10, also known as ubiquinone. It helps diabetics in much the same way as Vitamin E does by stimulating insulin production. The recommended dosage is 80 mg a day for approximately 3 months. Diabetics should notice stabilization in their blood sugar levels after this time.

Amino Acids

Diabetics who take amino acid supplements supply their body with some of the raw material needed for the manufacture of insulin, which is made up of 51 amino acids.

Digestive Enzymes

Diabetics have a pancreas that is not functioning as it should. Taking digestive enzymes such as amylase, protease, and lipase will assist diabetics in the absorption and digestion of nutrients.

The Diabetes Herb Treatment

Botanical herbs were used to treat diabetes long before insulin existed as an option. Over the last 20 years numerous studies have been done to show that many of the preparations used are extremely effective. I will only discuss the plants that have proven to be most effective in the treatment of diabetes. It is important to note that the treatment of diabetes requires a combination of different therapies and treatments. The use of botanical medicine serves to enhance treatment when combined with diet therapy, supplements, lifestyle etc;

Here are details about some of the botanical herbs used in the treatment of diabetes:

Bitter Melon

This is a tropical fruit that grows in South America, Asia and Africa. It resembles a cucumber and is covered in little bumps. Bitter melon is used as both a vegetable and a remedy for diabetes. Fresh juice that is extracted from the vegetable has proven to significantly lower blood sugar levels in type 2 diabetics. When injected like insulin, bitter melon has much the same effect with fewer side effects. Some diabetics use this herb as a replacement for insulin.

Onion (Allium Cepa) and Garlic (Allium Sativum)

Both onions and garlic are very helpful in lowering blood sugar levels. They contain Diallyl Disulphide Oxide (allicin) and Allyl Propyl Disulphide (APDS) which both effectively regulate blood circulation. Onions are a great source of chromium, which the body utilizes for insulin sensitivity and glucose metabolism.

According to Dr. Sarah Brewer the allicin found in garlic "prevents cells from taking up cholesterol, reduces cholesterol production in the liver and hastens the excretion of fatty acids, which in turn discourages atherosclerosis."

She also explained that garlic could play a role in preventing coronary heart disease since it helps to "reduce high blood pressure, lower levels of LDL cholesterol and triglycerides, reduce blood stickiness and improve the circulation."

Diabetics can liberally consume both garlic and onions since they are both extremely beneficial.

Salt Bush

Many years ago researchers did studies on sand rats to discover what effect salt bush has on diabetes. Sand rats usually eat a diet that consists mainly of salt bush. Several of the rats had their diet replaced by rat chow. Over time researchers found that they had developed very severe diabetes. When their diet was changed back to salt bush their condition improved dramatically.

This woody shrub found in North Africa, Southern Europe and the Mediterranean is sure to improve blood glucose regulation and glucose tolerance in type 2 diabetics. This is because it is full of protein, fiber, trace mineral and chromium. A dosage of 3 grams per day is enough to make a difference.

Gymnema Sylvestre

The Asian name for Gymnema Sylvestre is gurmar which means "sugar destroyer." This is a good indication of the effects that this herbal medicine has on glucose levels in the body. Gymnema's role in helping diabetics is twofold. It helps curb appetites, especially the appetites of those who crave sweet things. It also improves glucose control and has been shown to help with the regeneration of beta cells in the pancreas.

Type 1 diabetics who take Gymnesyl regularly might find that they can reduce their insulin intake after a while. It is also helpful to type 2 diabetics. In the past some type 2 diabetics managed to stop taking drugs as they were able to control blood sugar with Gymnesyl alone. A dosage of 200 mg twice a day or 400 mg once a day is recommended.

Bilberry

Also known as the European blueberry, this is a small deciduous shrub found in the woods and forests of Europe. Bilberries are full of nutrients and other beneficial substances that have proven to help diabetics. They contain an anthocyanoside known as myrtillin which helps lower blood glucose levels. Bilberry extracts have also proven to help improve circulation by strengthening blood vessels.

Diabetics who have developed diabetic retinopathy should seriously consider taking bilberry. Dr. Sarah Brewer explains: "It's benefits as a treatment for problems with vision arise from the antioxidant blue-red pigments it contains, which protect the membranes of light-sensitive and other cells in the eyes, reduce hardening and furring up of blood vessels, stabilize tear production, increase blood flow to the retina, and regenerate the light-sensitive pigment rhodopsin in the retina."

The recommended dosage of bilberry is between 20 and 60 dried ripe fruits or alternatively between 80 and 160 mg of dry extract daily.

Huereque

This is a herb derived from the root of the huereque cactus and is very effective in lowering blood sugar levels. A man by the name of Danie Dunphy once did a study on the effects of Huereque on 15 patients with adult onset diabetes. After a few months all of them were able to completely stop taking insulin.

Stevia

This herbal sweetener is effective in keeping blood sugar levels under control and does not need any insulin for its metabolism.

Fenugreek Seeds

This herb, found in the Mediterranean, India, and North Africa improves glucose control and lowers cholesterol levels. Studies done on Type 1 diabetics who took 50g of Fenugreek powder twice daily showed that their fasting blood sugar levels were lower and that there was a 54% reduction in the amount of glucose that was excreted through their urine.

Type 2 diabetics who took 15 grams of fenugreek powder noticed a significant decrease in their postprandial glucose levels.

Ginkgo Biloba

Also known as the maidenhair tree, Gingko Biloba is an old tree species whose leaves contain useful substances known as bilobalides and ginkgolidese. Extracts from the Ginkgo tree are helpful in improving and increasing circulation to different parts of the body including the brain. This increase in blood flow assists diabetics who struggle with impotence and Raynaud's disease, which is a condition that causes an interruption in blood flow to fingers and toes. Peripheral vascular insufficiency is common in diabetics so the increased blood flow to the peripheral tissues is one of the great benefits of taking Ginkgo biloba.

Gingko Biloba helps type 2 diabetics who have to take oral hypoglycemic drugs by increasing insulin secretion. In addition to that some studies have shown it to be useful as a blood thinning agent.

Additional Treatments for Diabetes

Exercise

The importance of exercise in the treatment of both NIDDM and IDDM simply cannot be emphasized enough. The improvements that will be seen in the diabetic who exercises regularly includes improved glucose tolerance, weight loss, greater insulin sensitivity, a reduction in total serum cholesterol and triglycerides, and ultimately a reduced need for exogenous insulin. It has been proven that regular exercise and weight loss reduce the risk of contracting diabetes by as much as 58 percent in those more prone to developing it. A simple 30 minute walk every day and adequate weight loss could make all the difference and could spare many people from having to suffer the often devastating effects of diabetes.

The reason why exercise is so beneficial to diabetics seems to lie in the fact that it causes chromium levels in the tissues to increase. Chromium is helpful in restoring insulin function and improving glucose tolerance.

It is recommended that diabetics try to exercise at least 3 times a week at an intensity that will raise their heart level by 50 percent for about 30 minutes.

Exercise is so beneficial to diabetics that it should certainly be a priority. It helps with weight loss, blood sugar control, oxygenation of tissues, and the stimulation of metabolic functions. When muscles are used vigorously the cells of the body absorb glucose that is used as energy without the help of insulin. This prevents the insulin surge that would usually be the body's response to sugar intake. It has been proven that Type 1 diabetics who exercise 3 to 4 times a week for 35-40 minutes will be able to reduce their need for insulin by as much as 25 percent.

It is important for diabetics to discuss their exercise plans and goals with their physician and to undergo a thorough cardiovascular examination. They also need to make sure that they properly monitor their blood sugar levels to avoid hypoglycemia.

Now before you get stressed about it, this is not about getting ready for iron man competitions or participating in the Olympics! Exercise is the most important contribution you can make to reaching and maintaining optimum physical health and prolonging life at any age.

In this case "exercise" is referring to activities that aim to help you relax and get rid of stress. This is the type of exercise that will take your mind off the problems in your life and help you to relax and enjoy each day. Exercise is something that should become a lifestyle – something that you can do every day. It doesn't need to be something that you stress and feel guilty about.

A Finnish study of nearly 8,000 men and women found that those who did not exercise increased their risk of death by 400% compared to individuals in the high-activity group.

There are lots of studies and much evidence that show how exercise helps to relieve tension, anxiety, depression, feelings of inadequacy and worries. It also improves mood, self-image, chronic constipation and increases energy.

Dr John Hibbs, N.D. of Bastyr University, in Kenmore, Washington says: "I don't think there's a single thing in life that is as therapeutic as the right kind of exercise program applied over time but misapplied, it can be just another stressor."

Evidently a tailored exercise program is worth investing in and committing to long-term.

Frequency and duration of activity are more important than the intensity with which you exercise. Moderately intense exercise such as brisk walking, is enough to benefit your health if done most days of the week. Normal daily activities as well as formal exercise sessions add up. You get health benefits from walking up stairs and carrying out the trash, doing the gardening, cleaning, shopping, vacuuming, making the bed, and mowing the lawn.

Remember: People who participate in regular exercise have a higher self-esteem, feel better, and are much happier than people who do not exercise. It has a mood-elevating effect and scientists say that is because it increases the level of endorphins, which are directly correlated with feeling good.

Remember This:

There are more than enough exercise regimes available for all people irrespective of age, abilities and/or disabilities. There is no excuse for not exercising.

Just do it.

Exercise Precautions

You need to make sure that you are in a condition to handle whatever you plan to do before you start. Here are a few practical guidelines to help you choose an exercise routine that you will enjoy and be able to do every day or very regularly.

- Consider your age

- Consider your current level of fitness, abilities and/or disabilities
- Consider the time of day that you will be able to do your exercises
- Consider how much time you have to do it

It is always recommended that you discuss your exercise plans with your physician, especially if you have not been active for some time. It is important to get a thorough physical check-up before you begin with any exercise regime. Tell your physician why you are having the check-up and what you plan to do since they may have some advice or input that will help you put the appropriate exercise plan together.

Everybody is aware of the fact that exercise is good for you. The problem is that for most of us the idea of having to join a gym and put ourselves through the physical grinder is totally unappealing. People don't always think in simple terms when it comes to exercising - they think it always means blood, sweat and tears. Nothing can be further from the truth; exercise need not be painful, stressful or expensive. My philosophy is that you should be able to enjoy it and be able to (actually want to) do it for the rest of your life.

Chelation therapy

Chelation therapy is a therapy that is done by administering chelating agents intravenously to remove heavy metals from the body. Diabetics have resorted to this form of treatment for many years to reduce and prevent complications. In the words of Dr. Gordon, M.D, of Payson Arizona:

"Over 20 years of clinical experience has shown that people with diabetes who receive intravenous EDTA chelation therapy have fewer amputations, less blindness, less kidney dialysis, and other complications of diabetes than those on conventional treatments,"

A study was done on 32 diabetic patients who had abnormally high levels of iron in their blood. A doctor by the name of Paul Cutler, M.D. chelated them with a chelating agent known as deferoxamine. The result was that 24 of them could completely stop taking their medication after 8-13 weeks. Dr. Cutler now firmly believes that deferoxamine could cure a third of all adult diabetics.

Oxygen Therapy

Oxygen therapy is used to treat both major and secondary complications of adult-onset diabetes. A lot of the problems that diabetics develop over time are linked to the circulation problems which have left the tissues in their body oxygen depleted. These problems include heart disease, diabetic neuropathy, vision loss, and gangrene.

Oxygen therapy introduces much needed oxygen into the diabetic's blood which helps to dramatically improve circulation and to enhance cellular metabolism. Once all the tissues in the body are receiving sufficient oxygen the body's processes will start running more smoothly.

Traditional Chinese Medicine

Traditional Chinese medicine is a combination of therapies that has been used to treat various illnesses for thousands of years. Over time it has become more sophisticated with its coherent and well developed approach to treatment. Some therapies in traditional Chinese medicine include acupuncture, diet therapy, mind/body exercise, Chinese massage, and various Chinese herbal medicines.

For many years traditional Chinese medicine has been used to treat diabetes. It is only helpful to type 1 diabetics if it is started in the early stages. Type 2 diabetics can consider this form of treatment during the beginning and intermediate stages of their condition. The approach of traditional Chinese practitioners differs to those of the Western world in that they don't constantly monitor and measure blood glucose levels in patients. Instead, they focus on treating the symptoms that manifest.

Acupuncture is a very important part of the treatment and the goal is to ultimately normalize endocrine function and reduce blood glucose levels. Studies have proven this to be very effective in many cases.

The use of Herbal medicine is an integral part of treating diabetes. Many herbs are used that are sourced from plants, animal parts, and minerals. Herbal remedies are prescribed to patients based on what symptoms they have whether it is excessive thirst, frequent urination, fatigue etc; Here is a list of some of the most common herbs used to treat diabetes. They help lower blood glucose levels and improve other symptoms but are most effective in helping diabetics utilize and process carbohydrates more effectively.

- Momodica Charantia – This herb is also referred to as "balsam pear" and is used to reduce blood glucose levels.
- Lagenaria Siceraria – Also known as "bitter gourd," this herb also helps to reduce blood glucose levels.
- Panax Ginseng - This herb has been used as a hypoglycaemic agent for a very long time and has been shown to lower blood glucose levels and improve the general mood of physiological state of diabetes patients.

- Psidium Gnajava – This herb is drunk as tea or taken in the form of fresh leaves and helps to lower blood glucose levels.

Diet therapy is another important part of the treatment utilized in TCM. Patients are usually evaluated based on their age, vitality, body type, geographic location, and seasonal influences in the process of prescribing a certain diet. A lot of attention is given to the amount and quality of food as well as how it is prepared and when exactly it is eaten. Patients are encouraged to eat small meals frequently and to eat seasonal foods instead of large amounts of sugar or fruits. Dr. Maoshing Ni, PhD. Maintains that diabetes is "an exhaustion syndrome caused by overindulging in sweet, fatty foods and wearing out the body," TCM aims improve the way the body functions as a whole by incorporating diet changes, herbs, massage, acupuncture, and acupressure.

Ayurvedic Medicine

Ayurvedic treatment for diabetes involves several steps including diet modification, panchakarma, exercise and herbal remedies.

The diabetic's diet is modified by reducing the intake of sugar, complex carbohydrates, protein and fat. They are encouraged to eat plenty of fresh vegetables, lemons, oranges, bitter fruits and herbs. The second step, panchakarma, is a cleansing program that is used to clear the auto antibodies which are antibodies that are against pancreatic tissue. This process includes a herbal steam sauna, herbal massages, and fasting. Thereafter the patient is subjected to a herbal purge to help cleanse the spleen, liver, and pancreas. Finally, they undergo colon therapy to clean out their digestive tract.

Exercise in the form of breathing exercises, physical exercise and yoga is strongly recommended to those undergoing Ayurvedic treatment. Ayurvedic practitioners make use of many different herbal remedies in their treatment of diabetes including turmeric capsules, lemon juice, bitter gourd, rose apple stones, fenugreek and amlaki powder. These herbal remedies have been shown to decrease the need for insulin and also lower blood sugar.

20 Recipes for Breakfast, Lunch Dinner and Snacks

Being diagnosed with diabetes certainly doesn't mean you need to brace yourself for a lifetime of tasteless, boring dishes! There are countless delicious recipes available to diabetics.

Below are some recipes which you can try and which will help you control your diabetes without having to starve or settle for bland and tasteless food. All of the recipes have been tried and tested and I can promise you they are really delicious.

To make it easy for you we have grouped the recipes into the various main meals and snacks.

5 Breakfast Options to Start Your Day

Turkey Sausage and Scrambled Eggs on a muffin

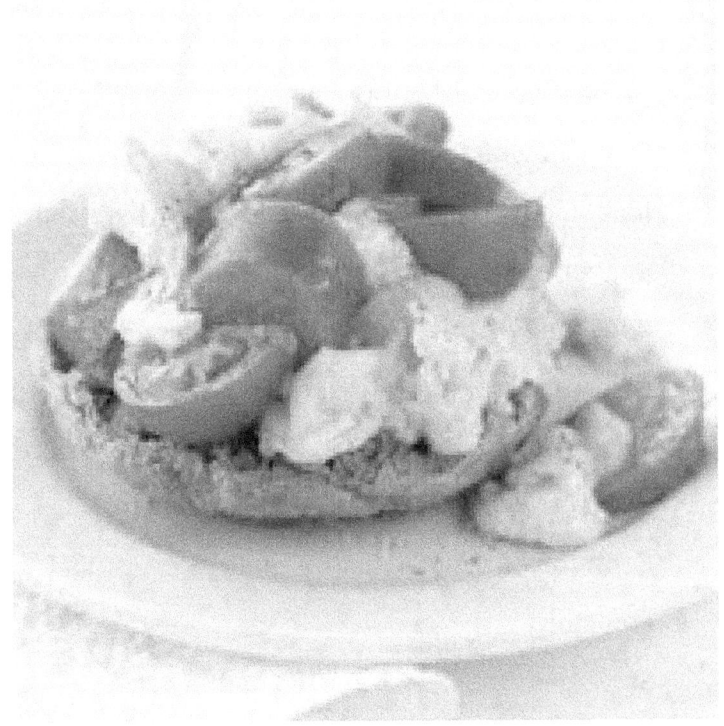

Ingredients

- Cooking Spray (non-stick)
- A pinch of ground black pepper
- 2 eggs
- 2 tbsp sodium reduced chicken broth
- 30g sliced turkey sausage
- 2 tbsp grated low fat cheddar cheese

- 1 toasted whole grain muffin
- ¼ cups diced cherry tomatoes

Preparation

1. Preheat your skillet over medium heat after you have coated it with the non-stick cooking spray.

2. In a medium bowl mix the eggs, broth, and black pepper and then stir in sliced sausage.

3. Pour the mixture into the heated skillet and cook over medium heat. Don't stir until the mixture begins to set.

4. Once the egg mixture is cooked add the cheese and tomatoes.

5. Cook for one more minute until the eggs look glossy and moist.

6. Serve the egg on your toasted muffin halves.

Oatmeal with Berries, Apples and Pecans

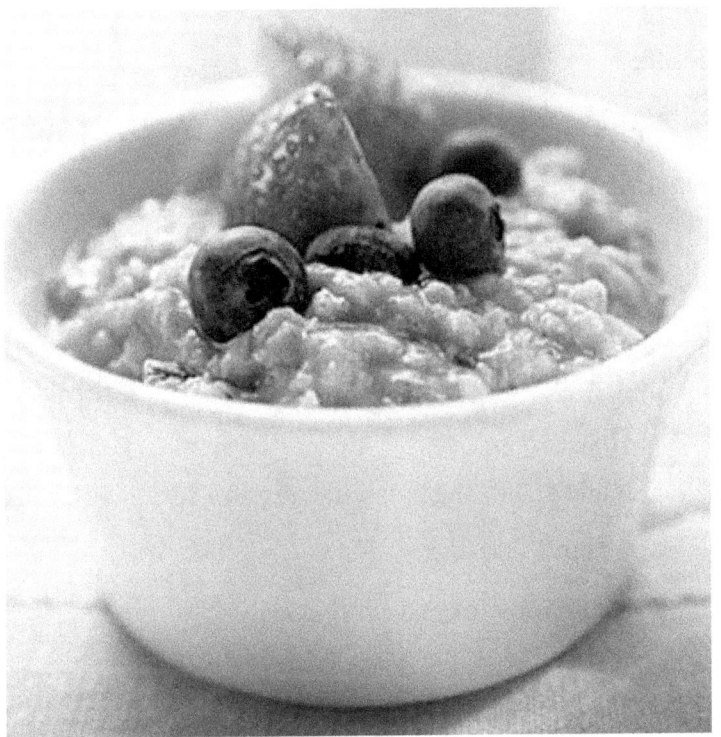

Ingredients

- 1cup oatmeal
- 2 cups water
- 1 ¾ cups apple juice
- 1 medium cored chopped apple
- ¼ teaspoon salt
- ½ teaspoon apple pie spice
- ½ cup blueberries, raspberries, or blackberries
- 1cup fat-free milk

- ¼ cup chopped almonds or pecans

Preparation

1. Combine the water and apple juice and bring to the boil in a large saucepan.

2. Stir in the oats, salt, apple and apple pie sauce.

3. Reduce heat and simmer uncovered for 30 minutes until the oats are cooked and have reached preferred consistency

4. Finally stir in the fresh berries and serve with milk and pecans if you like.

5. This recipe makes 6 servings.

Low Fat Bran Muffins

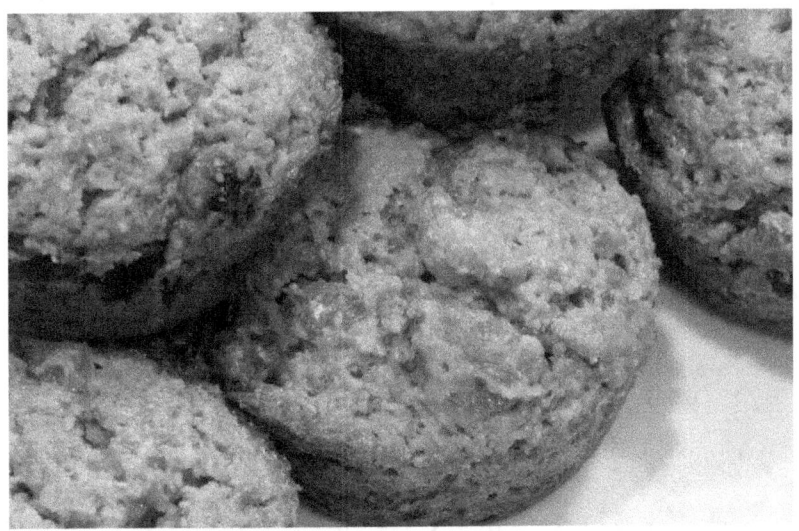

Ingredients

- 1 Egg
- 3 tbsp canola oil
- ¼ cup low-fat buttermilk
- ¼ cup unsweetened applesauce
- ¼ cup non-fat dry milk
- 1.5 tsp baking soda
- 1.5 cups all-purpose flour
- ¾ cup of Splenda granular
- 1 tsp ground cinnamon
- 2 tbsp of dried raisins or currants
- 2 tbsp of flax seeds
- 1 cup wheat bran

Preparation

1. Once you have preheated the oven to 35 °F (175°C), liberally spray a non-stick spray all over the muffin pan and put paper liners in the muffin cups.

2. Using a wire whisk mix the oil, vanilla, salt, applesauce, dry milk, Splenda granular, buttermilk and egg together.

3. Once everything is properly blended you can then add the cinnamon, baking soda, and wheat bran and keep stirring until everything is nicely mixed.

4. Spoon the batter into the lined muffin cups and finish off by sprinkling something like bran flakes on the top.

5. Bake for approximately 20 to 25 minutes.

These muffins are great when served warm.

Ham Cheese and Broccoli Dish

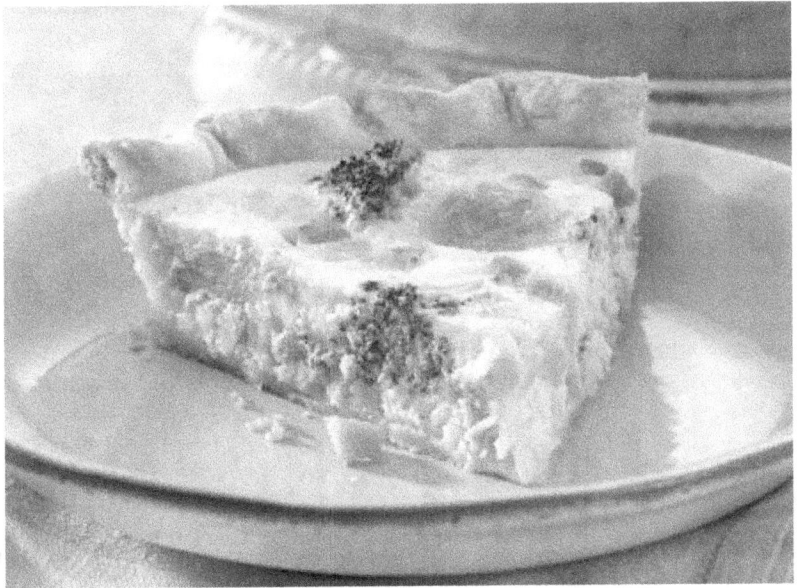

Ingredients

- 12 sheets phyllo dough (14 inches x 9 inches)
- 1 cup cubed cooked lean ham
- Refrigerated butter-flavored spray
- 1 package (16 ounces) frozen broccoli cuts that have been thawed
- 1 cup grated cheddar cheese (reduced fat)
- 1 small chopped onion
- 2 tbsp minced fresh parsley
- 2 minced garlic cloves
- 1/2 tsp dried thyme

- ½ tsp salt and ½ tsp pepper
- 1 cup egg substitute
- 1 cup fat-free evaporated milk
- 2 tbsp parmesan cheese (grated)

Preparation

1. Take one sheet of phyllo dough and spray with your butter-flavored spray. Place the finished product in a 9 inch pie dish that has been properly coated with cooking spray. One end of the dough should hang over the edge of the plate by approximately 3 inches. Repeat this process with the remaining dough and spray butter-flavored spray between each layer. (Remember to keep the dough covered with plastic wrap to ensure it doesn't dry out.)

2. Now combine the ham, cheese, broccoli, parsley, garlic, thyme, salt, pepper and onion in a large bowl and spoon the mixture into the crust. Now combine the milk and egg substitute and pour it over the broccoli mixture. The edges of dough should now be folded over towards the center of the pie dish. Spray the edges with the butter flavored spray

3. Now cover the edges of the crust with foil and bake at 374 degrees Fahrenheit (190 degrees Celsius) for 40

minutes. Then remove from the oven and take off the foil. Sprinkle with parmesan cheese and put the dish back in the oven for about 30 minutes. You will know it is ready when you insert a knife in the center and it comes out clean.

This recipe makes 6 servings.

Oatmeal Waffles

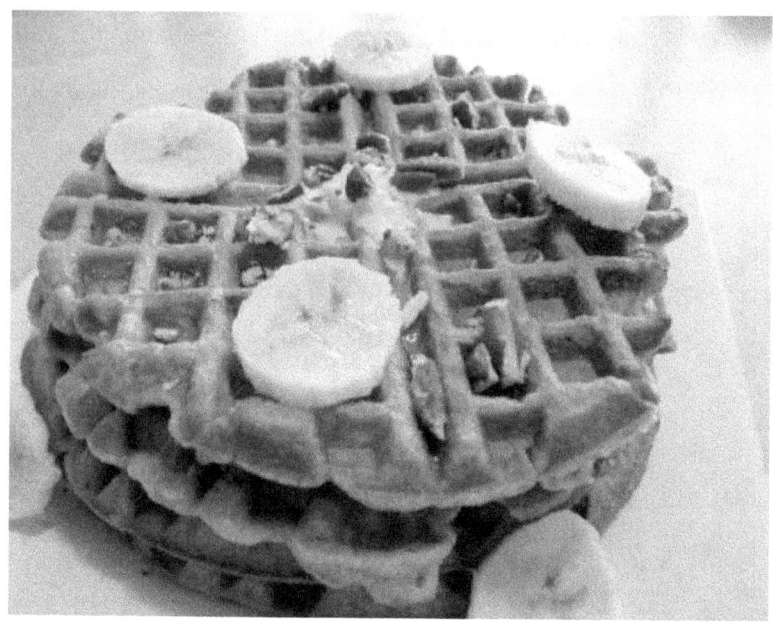

Ingredients

- 1 – 1/2 cups all-purpose flour
- 1 cup quick-cooking oats
- 3 tsp baking powder
- 1/2 teaspoon ground cinnamon
- 1/4 teaspoon salt
- 2 beaten eggs
- 1-1/2 cups milk
- 6 tbsp melted butter
- 2 tbsp Splenda

Preparation

1. Combine the flour, oats, baking powder, cinnamon and salt in a big bowl.

2. Take a smaller bowl and mix the milk, eggs, Splenda together.

3. Now combine the wet mixture with the dry mixture in the large bowl.

4. Grease the waffle iron and pour in the batter. Do not open until waffle is cooked.

5. Now top the waffle with yoghurt and fresh fruit.

6. This mixture makes 12 waffles.

Healthy Breakfast Shake

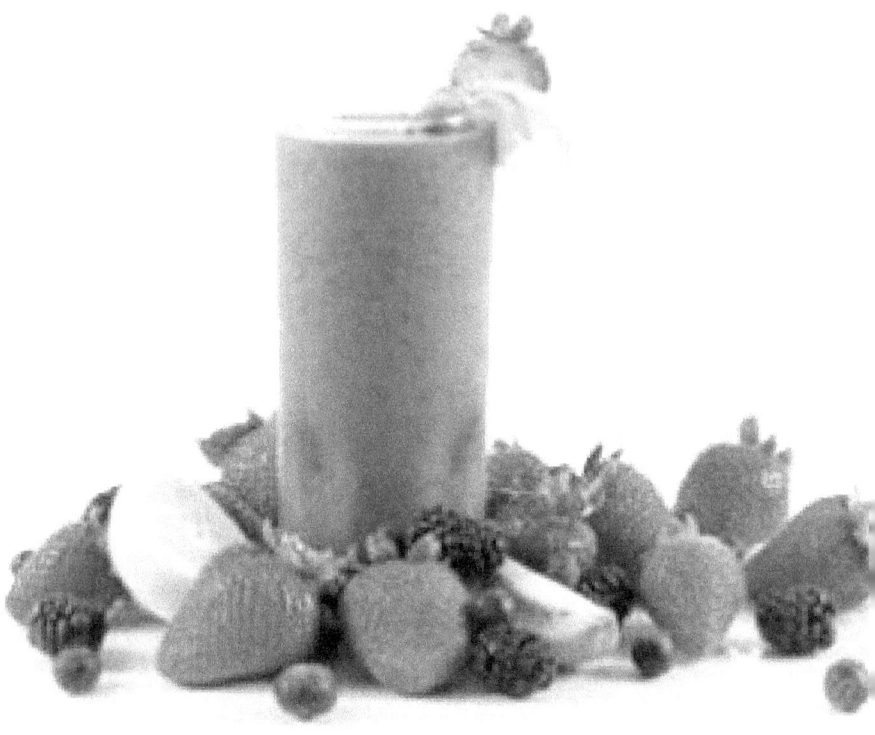

Some people prefer a lighter option for breakfast. If that is you, the breakfast shake/smoothie is a great alternative.

- Just blend 1 cup of skim milk with two of your favorite fruits.
- You could include a banana, 1 cup of strawberries, 1 tsp of wheat germ, 1 tsp of peanut butter etc.
- The possibilities are endless!
- To give your shake more substance, consider replacing the skim milk with non-fat yoghurt

5 Easy Lunch Meals

Chutney Chicken Wrap

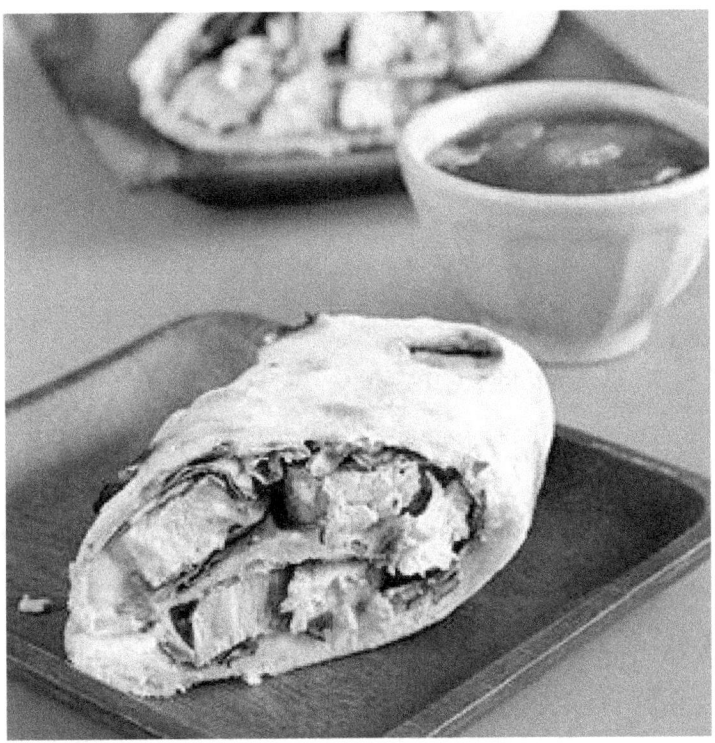

<u>Ingredients</u>

- 4 whole-wheat flour tortillas (8 to 9-inch rounds)
- 2 cups shredded coleslaw mix
- ¼ cup light or non-fat mayonnaise
- 1.5 tablespoons mango chutney
- 8 ounces roasted chicken or turkey breast (thinly sliced)
- 12 fresh spinach or lettuce leaves

Preparation

1. Combine the mayonnaise, chutney and coleslaw mix well.

2. Heat the tortillas and lay them on a flat surface.

3. Place a quarter of the chicken or turkey over half of one of your tortillas and top with ¼ of the coleslaw and the spinach/lettuce

4. Fold in the left and right margins in and then finish by rolling up each tortilla to enclose the filling.

5. Cut tortilla in half and serve.

Grilled Lamb Burgers

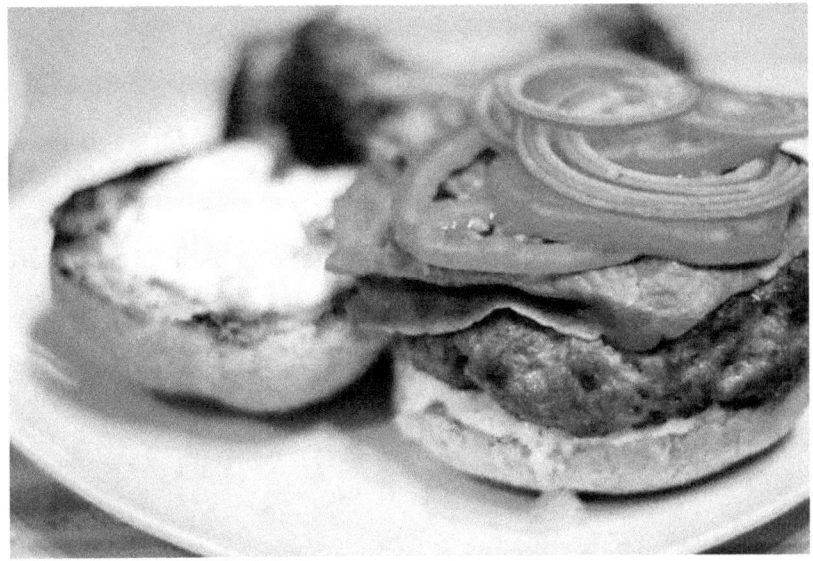

Ingredients

- pound of ground lamb meat
- ¾ teaspoon of fresh thyme minced
- finely chopped garlic cloves
- 1/4 teaspoon of fresh minced oregano
- 1 tablespoon of plain non-fat yogurt
- 1 tablespoon of lemon juice

Preparation

1. Prepare a gas grill by setting the heat to high or an outside grill by placing your oiled rack 4 inches above the coals.

2. Mix the meat with the thyme, garlic cloves, oregano non-fat yoghurt and lemon juice.

3. Form 4 patties out of the mixture.

4. Grill the burgers until they look perfect and ready for you. Here are some guidelines: 10 minutes for well done, 8 minutes for medium and 6 minutes for rare.

Chicken and Almond Salad with Rye Bread

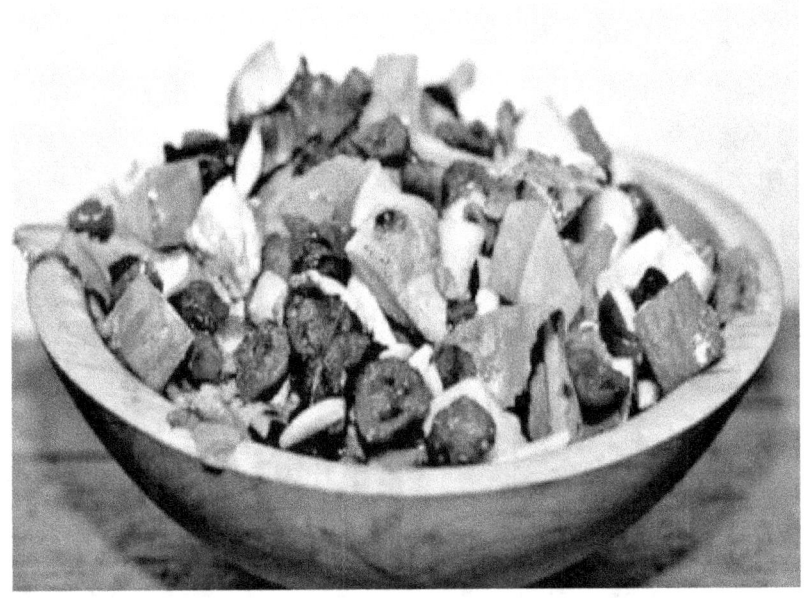

Ingredients

- 8 oz boneless skinless chicken breasts , cooked (cut into strips)
- 2 sliced celery stalks
- 2 tbsp fat free mayonnaise
- 1 tsp dried dill
- 1 tbsp slivered almonds
- pinch salt and black pepper
- 2 slices rye bread

Preparation

1. Chop chicken and celery. Place in a small bowl.

2. Toast almonds in oven and add to chicken.

3. Stir in mayonnaise, salt, pepper and dill.

4. Put the salad onto two separate plates and serve with rye bread.

Roast Beef Sandwich

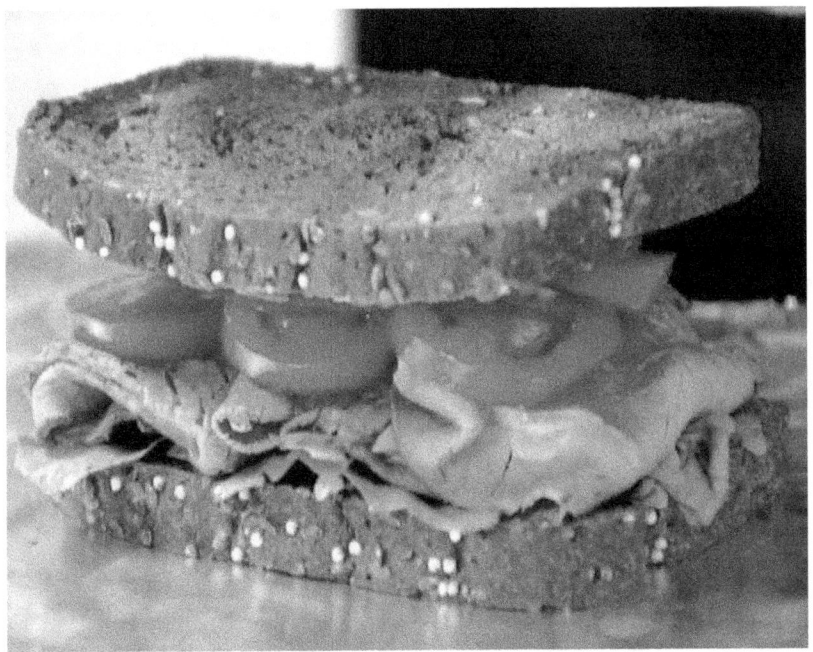

Ingredients

- 3 oz. roast beef, diced
- 2 tbsp. chopped celery
- 1/8 tsp. chopped chives
- 1/2 tbsp. lemon juice
- 1/2 med. tomato, chopped
- 1/2 tsp. salt
- 1/4 tsp. pepper
- 1 tsp. diet mayonnaise
- 2 slices thin bread

- Lettuce

Preparation

Combine all ingredients except bread and lettuce. Mix well. Spread on one slice of bread. Top with lettuce and remaining bread slice.

Turkey and Potato Salad

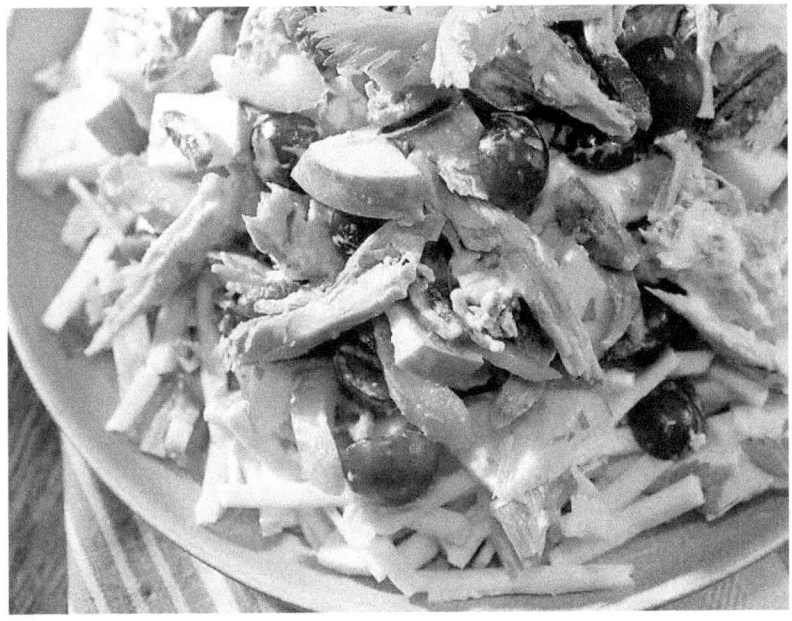

Ingredients

- 4 oz. cooked turkey or chicken, bite size pieces
- 1 (3 oz.) boiled potato, chopped
- 1 tbsp. mayonnaise
- 1 tsp. chopped pimento
- 1/2 tsp. dehydrated parsley flakes
- 1/2 tsp. nutmeg
- 1/2 tsp. sage
- 1/4 tsp. salt
- Dash of pepper
- Lettuce leaves

Preparation

Combine all ingredients except lettuce; mix well. Chill. Serve on lettuce leaves

5 Quick and Easy Meals for Dinner

Baked Garlic Chicken with Butter Beans

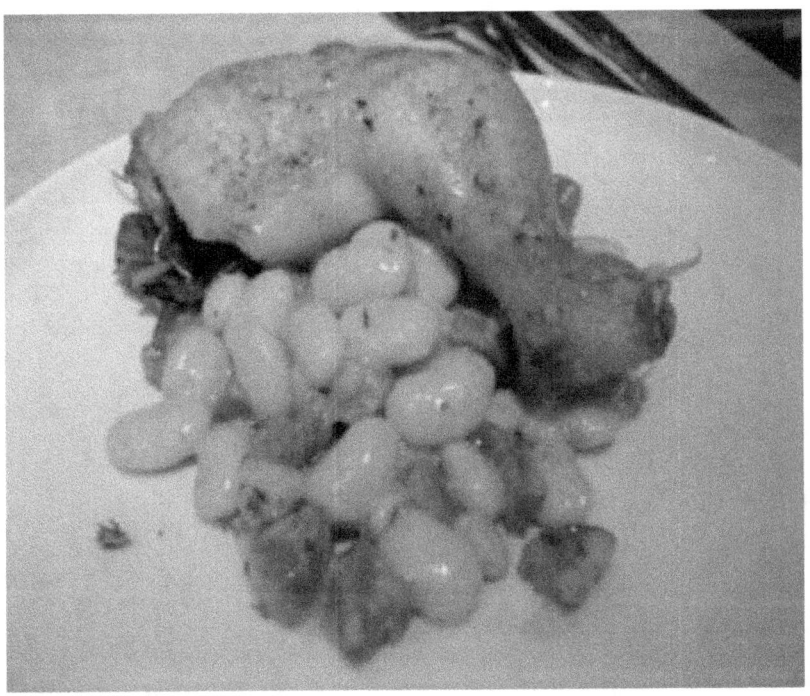

Ingredients

- 4 peeled garlic cloves
- 1 roughly chopped fennel bulb
  - pounds of chicken
- 2 handfuls of fresh parsley
- 2 x 14 ounces (400 g) cans of butter beans (drained)
- 1 ¼ cups of white wine
- 1 ¼ cups of vegetable stock

- Selection of cooked green vegetable to serve along with the chicken

Preparation

1. Preheat your oven to 356 degrees Fahrenheit (180 degrees Celsius).

2. Once you have washed the leeks slice them into thick pieces. Then onto the fennel - remove the core and roughly chop the flesh.

3. Mix the garlic cloves, fennel, leeks, parsley and butter beans into a bowl.

4. Now spread the mixture onto the bottom of a large casserole dish and pour in the vegetable stock and white wine.

5. Place your whole chicken on top of the mixture and then proceed to bring to the boil over the stove.

6. Now transfer the casserole dish into the oven and bake for approximately 1 to 1.5 hours.

7. Garnish with parsley and serve with the cooked green vegetables.

Traditional Spaghetti and Meatballs

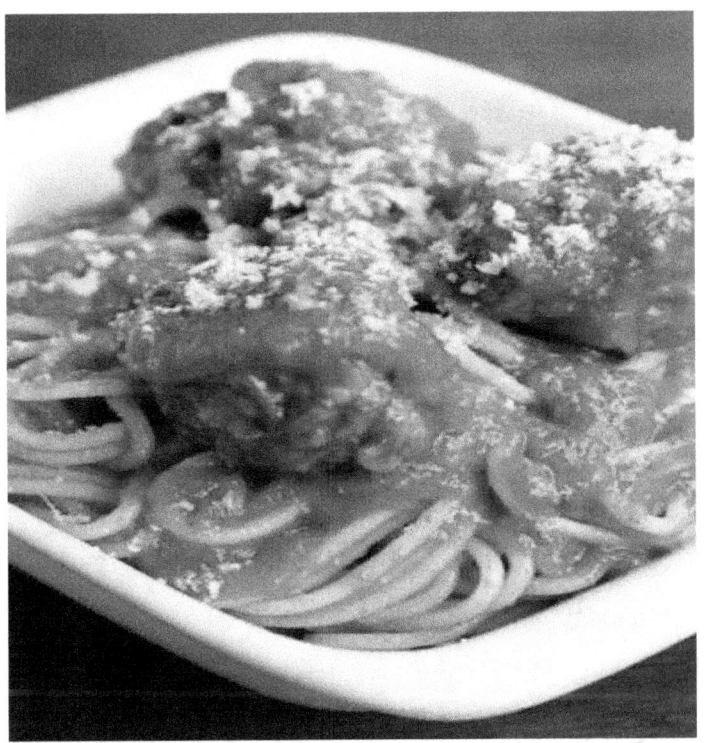

Ingredients

- 1 can undrained crushed tomatoes, 1 can tomato paste, 1 cup water, 1tsp dried oregano, ¾ cup chopped onion,

- 1 tbsp olive oil, 1 minced garlic clove, ½ teaspoon salt, ½ teaspoon pepper

- Meatballs: 4 slices bread broken into little pieces, 1/2 cup water, 2 eggs, lightly beaten, 1/2 cup Parmesan cheese grated, 1 garlic clove, minced, 1 teaspoon dried basil, 1 teaspoon dried parsley flakes, ½ teaspoon salt, 1 pound lean ground beef, 2 teaspoons olive oil, 1 package (16 ounces) spaghetti

Preparation

1. In a large saucepan sauté onions and garlic.
2. Combine the tomatoes, tomato paste, water, oregano, salt and pepper and bring to the boil.
3. Reduce heat and allow simmering for 30 minutes.
4. Take bread and soak it in a bowl for 5 min.
5. Once that is done squeeze the liquid out of the bread and combine it with the cheese, eggs, garlic, basil, parsley, and salt.
6. Add the beef into the mixture and mix before forming 1 inch balls.
7. In a non-stick skillet brown meatballs in oil over medium heat.
8. Add meatballs to sauce and bring to a boil.
9. Reduce heat and simmer for approximately 30 minutes. You will know it is ready when the meatballs are no longer pink.
10. Cook spaghetti according to package directions and serve with meatballs.

Cashew Vegetable Stir Fry

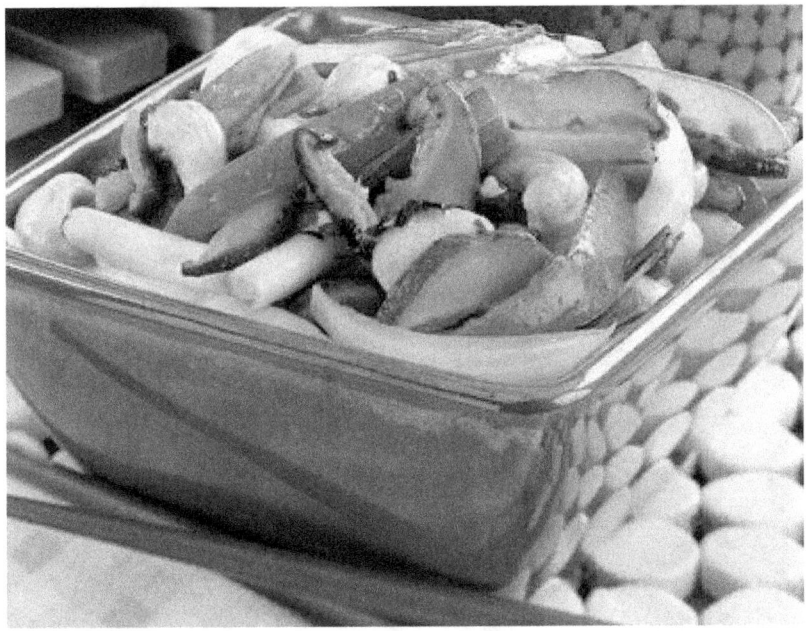

Ingredients

- 3 tablespoons of olive oil
- A selection of vegetables: About 2 pounds (900 grams) of a combination of mushrooms, carrots, baby sweetcorn, beansprouts, peppers, spring onions, and mangetouts
- 1 tablespoon of fresh root ginger
- 1 ½ cups of cashew nuts
- 4 tablespoons of pumpkin, sesame or sunflower seeds
- Soy sauce
- Black pepper and sea salt

Lamb Stew with a Middle Eastern Twist

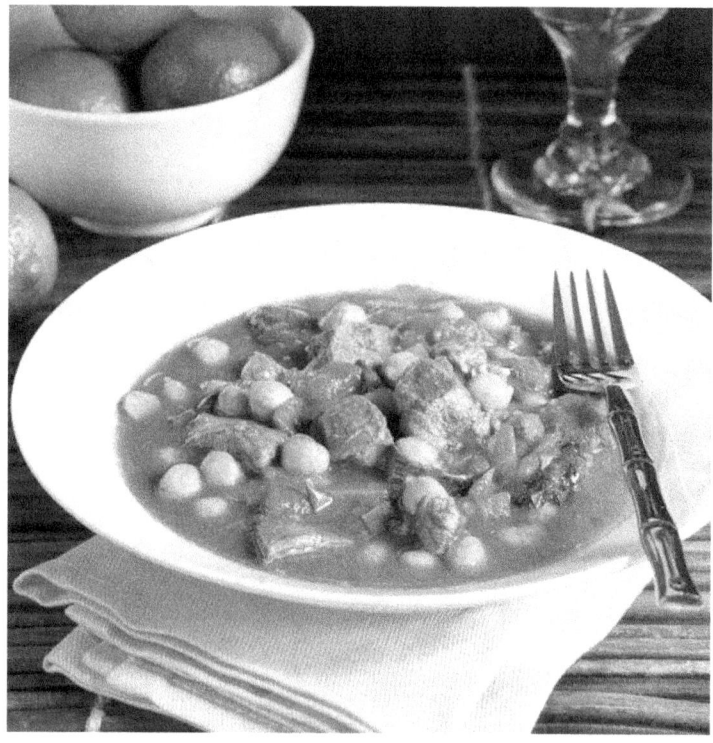

Ingredients

- 24 oz (680g) boneless lamb stew meat, preferably the shoulder cut
- ¼ tsp Salt
- Freshly ground pepper (as much as you like)
- 2 medium chopped onions
- 1 can diced tomatoes
- ¾ cup reduced-sodium chicken broth
- 1 tbsp olive or canola oil

- 4 tsp ground cumin
- 1 tbsp ground coriander
- ¼ tsp cayenne pepper
- 4 minced garlic cloves
- 1can chickpeas (rinsed)
- 6 oz baby spinach

Preparation

1. Combine oil, coriander, cumin, cayenne, salt and pepper in a bowl and set aside.

2. Now put the lamb in a slow cooker and coat with the spice mixture.

3. Finish off by placing onions in your dish.

4. Using a saucepan, bring the tomatoes, garlic and broth to a simmer over medium heat and proceed to pour over lamb.

5. Cover and cook until the lamb is very tender. This will require 3 to 3.5 hrs on high or 5.5 to 6 hrs on low heat.

6. Measure 1.5 cup of chickpeas and mash in a bowl. Stir the mashed chickpeas, along with the remaining whole chickpeas into your stew and also add the spinach.

7. Place in the over for another 5 min or until the spinach has wilted.

Shrimp Vegetable and Creamy Garlic Pasta

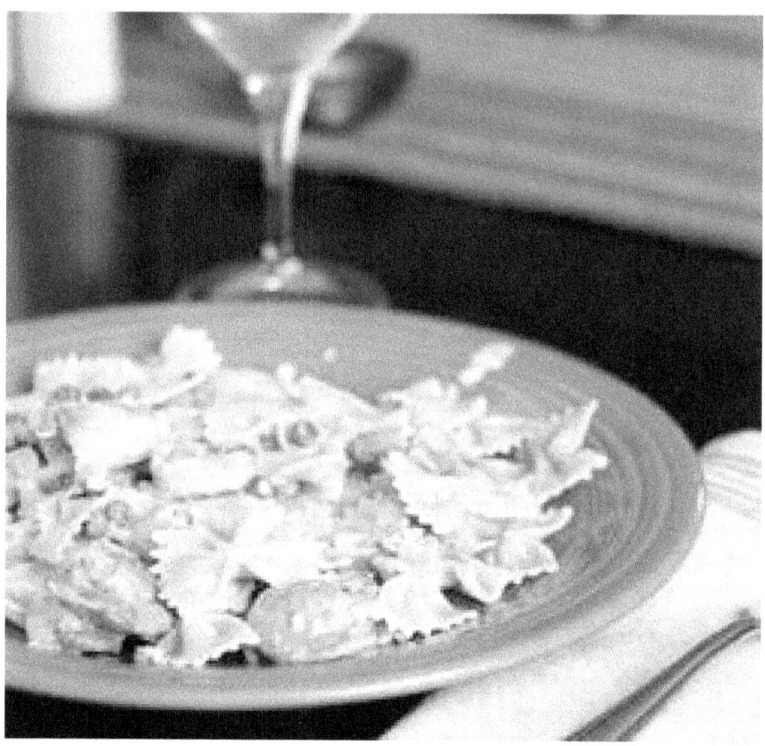

Ingredients

- 6 oz (170g) whole-wheat spaghetti
- 340g raw, peeled, deveined shrimp that has been cut into 1 inch pieces peeled and deveined raw
- 1 bunch trimmed asparagus – slice into thin pieces
- 3 cloves chopped garlic and 1 ¼ tsp kosher salt
- 1 1/2 cups low-fat or non-fat plain yoghurt
- 1 large red pepper – slice into thin pieces
- 3 tbsp lemon juice

- 1 tbsp extra-virgin olive oil
- ½ tsp freshly ground pepper
- 1 cup peas
- ¼ cup chopped flat-leaf parsley

Preparation

1. Bring a large pot of water to a boil.
2. Add spaghetti and cook according to package instructions.
3. Add bell pepper, shrimp, peas and asparagus. Cook until shrimp are pasta is cooked. This should take between 2 and 4 minutes.
4. Drain well.
5. Combine garlic and salt in a large bowl and mash into a paste.
6. Now using a whisk add the yogurt, lemon juice, parsley, pepper and oil.
7. Finally, add the delicious pasta mixture and toss.

5 Healthy Snacks for Anytime

Homemade Granola Bars

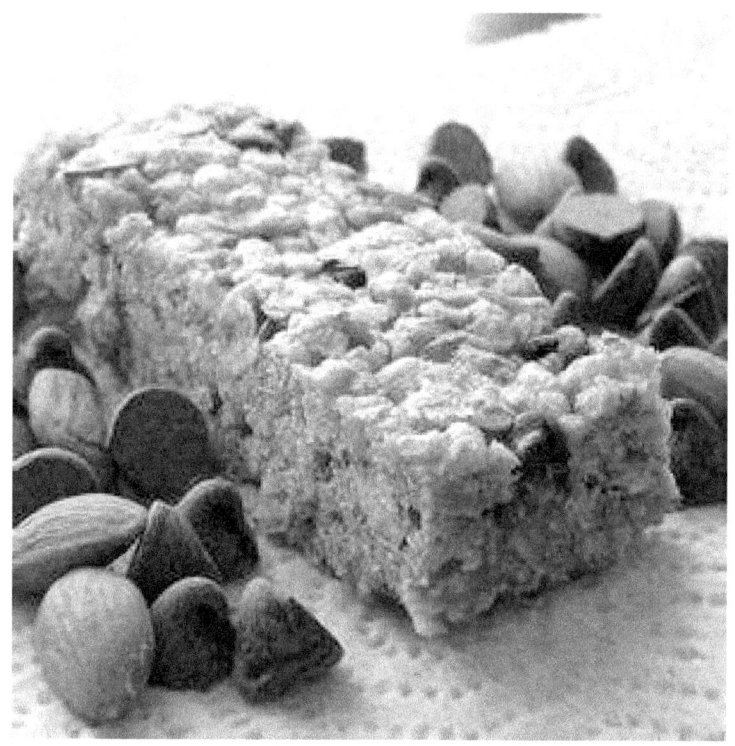

Ingredients

- 1 1/2 cups rolled gluten free oats
- 4 tbsp golden flax seeds
- 1 cup pumpkin seeds
- 2 tbsp sesame seeds
- ¾ cup dry, roasted and unsalted macadamia nuts
- ¾ cup dry, roasted unsalted almonds

- ¼ cup coconut oil

- ½ cup unsweetened coconut flakes

- ¼ cup natural agave nectar

Preparation

1. Preheat oven to 300 degrees F.

2. Combine the oats, nuts, seeds and coconut flakes

3. Combine the oil and agave nectar in a pot and heat over the stove until warm.

4. Combine the oat and oil mixture until properly mixed

5. Spread the mixture onto a large baking sheet

6. Put in the oven and bake for around 45 minutes. To prevent the mixture from sticking slide a spatula underneath every now and then. You will know your bars are ready when they are nice and crisp.

7. Allow them to cool before storing in sealed containers.

Delicious Cookies – Without the Sugar

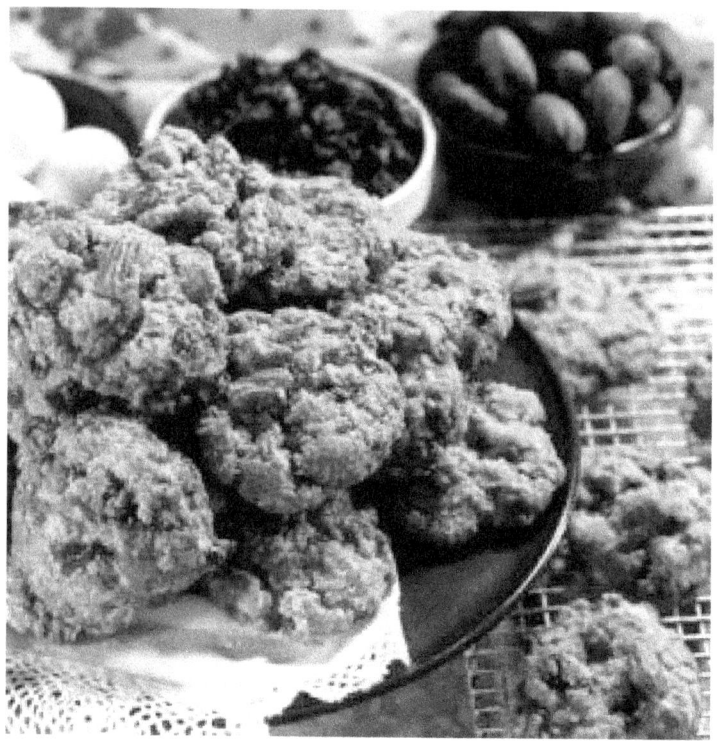

Ingredients

- 1 cup Raisins
- ¾ cup Shortening
- 2 Eggs
- 1 tsp. Vanilla
- 1 cup water
- 1 can frozen sugarless apple juice that has been thawed and diluted. Should make 1 ½ cups liquid.
- 3 cups flour

- ½ tsp. baking Powder

- Pinch of salt

- ½ cup chopped nuts

- 1 cup coconut

- 1 tsp. soda

- 1 tsp. cloves

- 2 tsp. cinnamon

Preparation

1. Combine the water and raisins and simmer for 15 minutes. Drain the juice and add water until you have ¾ cup.

2. Cream the shortening and eggs and then add the sugarless apple juice and mix well

3. Sift the baking powder, flour, soda, cinnamon, cloves and salt. Add the dry mixture to the egg mixture and beat well.

4. Now stir in the raisins and the ¾ cup of liquid, coconut and chopped nuts.

5. Spray a cookie sheet with Pam and place rounded tablespoons of the mixture onto the sheet.

6. Bake at 350 degrees Fahrenheit for 10-12 minutes.

Chewy Brownies

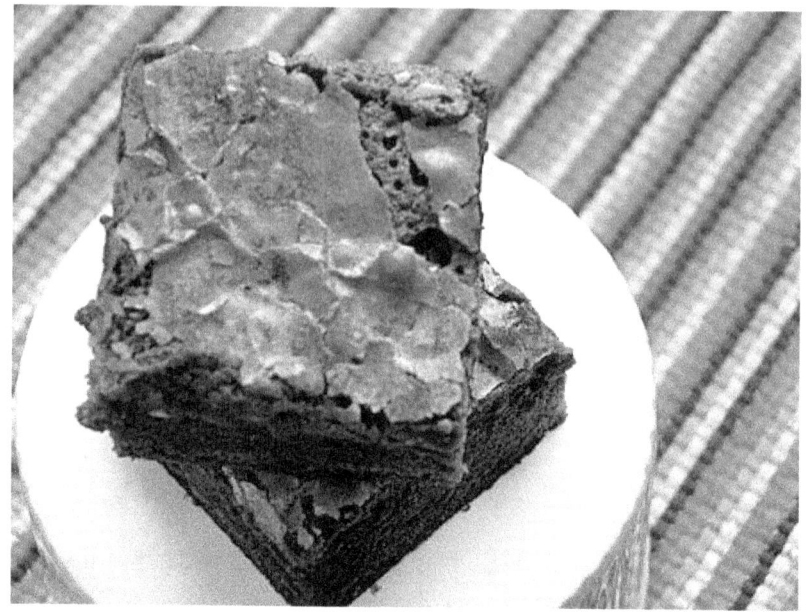

Ingredients

- 3/4 cup flour
- ½ cup butter
- ½ cup Splenda
- 2 eggs
- ½ tsp baking powder
- ½ tsp salt
- ½ cup chopped nuts
- 1 tsp vanilla
- 1 ½ squares chocolate (unsweetened)

Preparation

1. Melt the chocolate and butter in a saucepan over low heat. Once you have removed the mixture from the heat, blend and stir in the Splenda and vanilla and add eggs one at a time

2. Sift flour, baking powder and salt together and combine with chocolate mixture.

3. Pour the mixture into a greased pan and liberally sprinkle nuts over the top.

4. Bake at180 deg. Celsius for 25 minutes.

5. Before it has completely cooled cut into squares, preferably with a plastic knife as it is easier that way.

Peanut Clusters

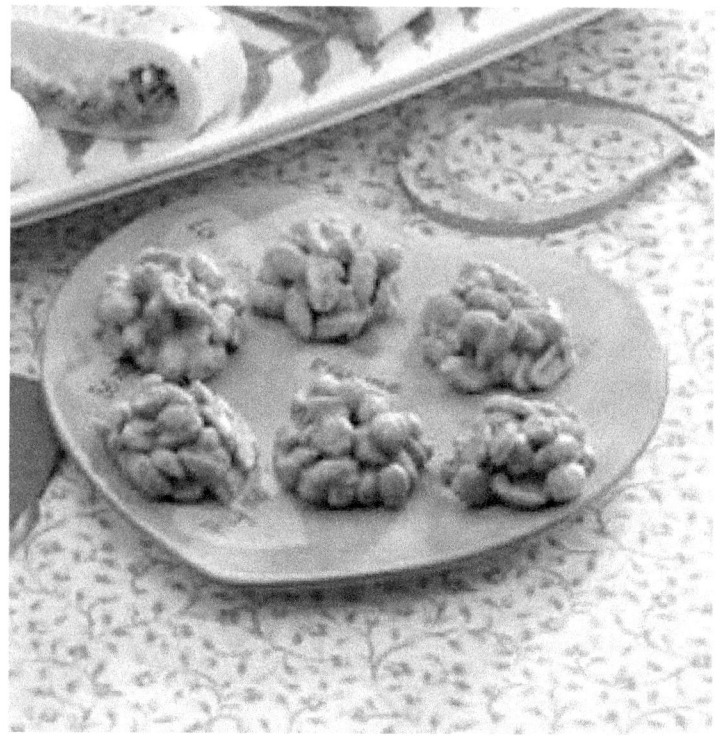

<u>Ingredients</u>

- 1/3 cup peanut butter
- 1 tbsp. honey
- ½ cup raisins
- ¼ cup dry roasted peanuts
- 1 tbsp cocoa powder
- 1 packet artificial sweetener
- 1/4 cup Grape Nuts cereal

Preparation

1. Melt honey and peanut butter on the stove (low heat). Once melted remove from heat and stir in the rest of the ingredients except for the cereal.

2. Scoop some of the mixture with a teaspoon and roll into cereal to form balls.

Pumpkin and Raisin Bars

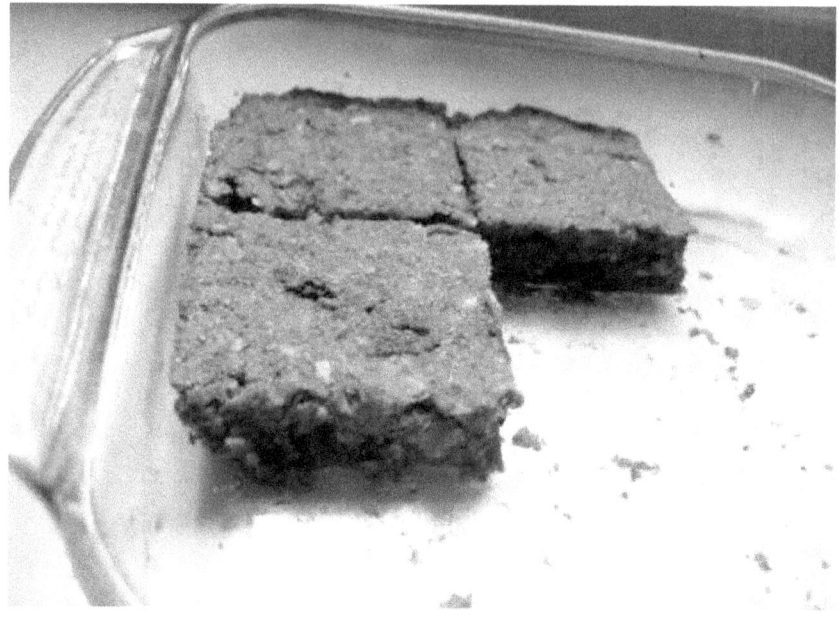

<u>Ingredients</u>

- 4 eggs
- 1 cups Splenda
- 2 tsp. cinnamon
- ½ tsp nutmeg
- 1 cup raisins
- 1 can pumpkin (15 oz.)
- ½ tsp ginger
- ¾ cup oil
- 2 cups flour
- 2 tsp. baking powder

- ½ tsp soda
- ½ tsp. salt

Preparation

1. In a large bowl combine the soda, baking powder, flour, salt and spices. In a separate bowl which the eggs until they are fluffy.
2. Gradually add Splenda into the eggs and be sure to beat well.
3. Now stir in the dry ingredients, pumpkin and raisins.
4. Grease your pan before the spread the batter evenly.
5. Bake for 30 – 35 minutes at 350 degrees Fahrenheit.
6. Allow to cool on a rack and frost with cream cheese frosting.

Fats: The Good, the Bad and the Ugly

There has always been a lot of confusion surrounding fat in the diet. What is good and what is bad? Some believe that all fats are bad and therefore need to be completely eliminated from the diet. That approach is not correct and is not based on science or good practice. There are good fats and there are bad fats and you need to know the difference.

In order to eliminate some of the confusion I have added an insert from the diet chapter in one of my other Kindle books "Heart Disease Prevention and Reversal."

Hopefully this information will clear up any misconceptions you might have and convince you of the importance of the good fats.

Good Fats and Bad Fats

At this stage it is probably important to understand that not all fats (oils) are created equal. Our bodies need fats because it helps with absorption of nutrients from our food, nerve transmission, maintenance of the cell membranes and many other vital functions.

Bad fats contribute to weight gain, inflammation, heart disease and cancer, while good fats promote a healthy body. It is therefore important to replace the bad fats with good fats in our diet.

The Good Fats

The good fats consist of 2 groups, Monounsaturated Fats and Polyunsaturated Fats.

Monounsaturated Fats

Monounsaturated fats are those fats that we find in most nuts; peanuts, almonds, walnuts and pistachios. We also encounter them in avocado, canola and olive oil. It has been proven that monounsaturated fats help in weight loss, lowering of total cholesterol and LDL cholesterol while increasing HDL cholesterol.

Polyunsaturated Fats

Polyunsaturated fats are encountered in seafood like salmon and fish oil. It has also been proven that Polyunsaturated fats lower total cholesterol and LDL cholesterol while it raises HDL cholesterol.

The Bad and the Ugly Fats

The bad fats consist of 2 groups, saturated fats and transfats.

Saturated Fats

Saturated fats are encountered in red meat, dairy, fatty beef, lamb, pork, poultry with skin, beef fat (tallow), lard and cream, butter, cheese and other dairy products made from whole or reduced-fat (2 percent) milk, eggs and seafood as well as some plant oils such as coconut oil, palm oil and palm kernel oil. It has been shown to raise total blood cholesterol as well as LDL cholesterol.

Saturated fats and transfats (from hydrogenated oils) create a serious risk for heart disease. In a study that tracked the medical conditions of 5,200 men (age 42-53) over a period of 22 years the finding was:

The men with higher blood levels of saturated fats and transfats were up to 70% more likely to experience sudden death form heart disease than the men with lower levels.

Trans Fats

Transfats are the real bad brother of the two. Certain oils are "hydrogenated" (hydrogen is added) in order to have a longer shelf life and are found in many of the commercially packaged foods, fried food such as French fries in fast food chains, packaged snacks such as microwaved popcorn as well as in vegetable shortening and margarine. Eating these types of foods poses a serious risk to our health, as you will see below.

It is a well-known fact that saturated and transfats increase the levels of LDL and therefore increase the risk of heart disease. More recently it was found that transfats are actually much worse than saturated fats.

29 healthy, non-smoking people were divided into 2 groups to follow a diet high in transfats (9.2% of total calories) for one group and the other group on a diet with the same amount of saturated fats. The findings were:

That the transfat diet reduced blood vessel function by 29% and also reduced healthy HDL levels by 20%, compared to the saturated-fat diet.

Omega Fatty Acids

These days there is also a lot of talk and hype about omega fatty acids and words like Omega 3, Omega 6 and Omega 9 are being thrown around every day.

What are Omega Fatty Acids?

Omega fatty acids are also called essential fatty acids. Essential because the body cannot produce Omega fatty acids and you have to provide it to your body through your diet. Note that only Omega 3 and 6 are essential, not Omega 9, because our body can actually manufacture Omega 9. The omega fatty acids are vital for your body functions in order to maintain cellular health, prevent inflammation, maintain the nervous system and fight certain illnesses.

Many studies have shown that Omega fatty acids can prevent cancer, help with mental health disorders, lower LDL cholesterol, raise HDL cholesterol and many other benefits.

There are three different kinds of Omega fatty acids; Omega 3, 6, and 9. Each of them has a different chemical structure therefore the different numbers 3, 6 and 9.

Omega 3

Omega 3 fatty acids are in oily fishes and in fish oil supplements. Omega 3s have been shown to help prevent and cure heart disease (see studies below), lower high blood pressure, fight inflammation, assist those with arthritis and other autoimmune disorders and help with mental disorders and improve people with ADD and ADHD as well.

Omega-3 fatty acids are the most important of the three fatty acids. The most important reason for this is because they suppress inflammation, which is the cause of many of the degenerative diseases, including heart disease.

In order to lower the level of homocysteine it is of vital importance that you complement your diet with essential fatty acids (EFAs) which is found in the Omega-3 oils from flaxseed oil, ocean algae or from cold saltwater fish, such as Scandinavian salmon, orange roughly, halibut and other types of fish and seafood. These oils are extremely useful in reducing LDL cholesterol and have proved to prevent heart attacks by eliminating clotting and arterial damage.

Omega 6

Omega 6 fatty acids are in plant sources like nuts and flax seeds. These essential fatty acids have many of the same benefits as Omega 3. It has been shown to reduce inflammation and help people with arthritis and other autoimmune diseases, have very positive effects on skin diseases such as acne and psoriasis. It is also very helpful in the prevention and treatment of heart disease (see studies below).

It is very important that we try to balance the ratio of intake of Omega 3 to Omega 6. Most of us get too much Omega 6 in our diets. Omega 6 can be found plentifully in many vegetable cooking oils such as soybean oil, sunflower oil, canola oil and corn oil (but not olive oil). They're also common ingredients in many of the foods we consume, which is why most of us have a heavily imbalanced ratio of Omega-6's to 3's.

Omega 6 prevents the stickiness of blood platelets, allowing blood to pass through the arteries without danger of clotting. The best sources of Omega 6 are borage oil, black currant oil, and evening primrose oil and grapeseed oil, which contain 76% linoleic acid (an omega-6 oil). Grapeseed oil has a high concentration of vitamin E, a vital antioxidant.

Omega 9

This is the lesser-known fatty acid of the three. However Omega 9 does play a large role in a healthy body. On the other hand it is the most abundant fatty acids of all in nature and is not in short supply in our diets. They are also not considered essential because our bodies can make Omega-9 from unsaturated fat.

The best source of Omega 9 is olive oil. Olive oil has been shown to be an extremely effective preventer of disease but this is mainly due to the high polyphenol content rather than to its fatty acid content.

Olive oil should be used for all cooking because of its strong antioxidant, anti-inflammatory, anti-clotting and antibacterial effects.

Omega 9 is also found in animal fat other vegetable oils and avocados and does play a vital role in cancer prevention and heart protection; however these should generally make up a smaller part of your diet because they can include saturated fats, which are harmful to the heart in larger quantities.

Getting More Essential Fatty Acids in Your Diet

The best sources of essential fatty acids are – fish, flaxseed, avocados, olive oil, grapeseed oil, nuts etc. You should make sure that you have healthy servings of those in order to maintain a healthy body and heart.

Things have been made much easier with the availability of all the Omega fatty acids in supplement form. These supplements are usually in a capsule form and are easy to take, easy to digest and easy to remember.

The Diabetic's Shopping List

For diabetics it is critical to follow a diet high in complex carbohydrates and fiber. Below are a few suggestions of what you should be putting in your shopping basket/trolley from now on.

1. Fiber rich foods such as coarse 100% whole-grain breads and minimally processed whole-grain cereals, oats, nuts, seeds, apples, pears, and beans. Aim to consume at least 50 grams of fiber daily.

2. Complex carbohydrate foods (with low GI as in the next chapter) which will include most fresh vegetables, most legumes, and most nuts, green peas, orange carrots, red tomatoes, all leafy greens, sweet potatoes and yams, pitted fruits and melons as well as brown rice.

3. Protein and dairy should consist of skim milk, buttermilk, poultry, lean cuts of beef, pork, and veal, shellfish and white-fleshed fish.

Don't Buy this

Here is what you should not put in your shopping basket/trolley: White bread, bagels, English muffins, packaged flaked cereals, instant hot cereals, low-fat frozen desserts, dried fruits, whole milk and whole-milk cheeses, hot dogs, and luncheon meats.

- Avoid eating any refined sugar.
- Never eat "junk food."
- Be sure to include protein snacks in your diet between meals.
- Pack your diet with complex carbohydrates.
- Reduce the amount of alcohol, caffeine, and tobacco you take in.

Glycemic Index

Information provided by the University of Sydney and used with permission.

Breakfast Cereal

Low GI		Medium GI		High GI	
All-bran (UK/Aus)	30	Bran Buds	58	Cornflakes	80
All-bran (US)	50	Mini Wheats	58	Sultana Bran	73
Oat bran	50	Nutrigrain	66	Branflakes	74
Rolled Oats	51	Shredded Wheat	67	Coco Pops	77
Special K (UK/Aus)	54	Porridge Oats	63	Puffed Wheat	80
Natural Muesli	40	Special K (US)	69	Oats in Honey Bake	77
Porridge	58	Medium GI		Team	82
		Bran Buds	58	Total	76
				Cheerios	74
				Rice Krispies	82
				Weetabix	74
				Cornflakes	80

Staples

Low GI		Medium GI		High GI	
Wheat Pasta Shapes	54	Basmati Rice	58	Instant White Rice	87
New Potatoes	54	Couscous	61	Glutinous Rice	86
Meat Ravioli	39	Cornmeal	68	Short Grain White Rice	83
Spaghetti	32	Taco Shells	68	Tapioca	70
Tortellini (Cheese)	50	Gnocchi	68	Fresh Mashed Potatoes	73
Egg Fettuccini	32	Canned Potatoes	61	French Fries	75
Brown Rice	50	Chinese (Rice) Vermicelli	58	Instant Mashed Potatoes	80
Buckwheat	51	Baked Potatoes	60		
White long grain rice	50	Wild Rice	57		
Pearled Barley	22				
Yam	35				
Sweet Potatoes	48				
Instant Noodles	47				
Wheat tortilla	30				

Bread

Low GI		Medium GI		High GI	
Soya and Linseed	36	Croissant	67	White	71
Wholegrain Pumpernickel	46	Hamburger bun	61	Bagel	72
Heavy Mixed Grain	45	Pita, white	57	French Baguette	95
Whole Wheat	49	Wholemeal Rye	62		
Sourdough Rye	48				
Sourdough Wheat	54				

Snacks & Sweet Foods

Low GI		Medium GI		High GI	
Slim-Fast meal replacement	27	Ryvita	63	Pretzels	83
Snickers Bar (high fat)	41	Digestives	59	Water Crackers	78
Nut & Seed Muesli Bar	49	Blueberry muffin	59	Rice cakes	87
Sponge Cake	46	Honey	58	Puffed Crispbread	81
Nutella	33			Donuts	76
Milk Chocolate	42			Scones	92
Hummus	6			Maple flavoured syrup	68
Peanuts	13				
Walnuts	15				
Cashew Nuts	25				
Nuts and Raisins	21				
Jam	51				
Corn Chips	42				

Legumes (Beans)

Low GI		Medium GI		High GI	
Kidney Beans (canned)	52	Beans in Tomato Sauce	56		
Butter Beans	36				
Chick Peas	42				
Haricot/Navy Beans	31				
Lentils, Red	21				
Lentils, Green	30				
Pinto Beans	45				
Blackeyed Beans	50				
Yellow Split Peas	32				
Kidney Beans (canned)	52				
Butter Beans	36				

Vegetables

Low GI		Medium GI		High GI	
Frozen Green Peas	39	Beetroot	64	Pumkin	75
Frozen Sweet Corn	47			Parsnips	97
Raw Carrots	16				
Boiled Carrots	41				
Eggplant/Aubergine	15				
Broccoli	10				
Cauliflower	15				
Cabbage	10				
Mushrooms	10				
Tomatoes	15				
Chillies	10				
Lettuce	10				
Green Beans	15				
Red Peppers	10				
Onions	10				

Fruits

Low GI		Medium GI		High GI	
Cherries	22	Mango	60	Watermelon	80
Plums	24	Sultanas	56	Dates	103
Grapefruit	25	Bananas	58		
Peaches	28	Raisins	64		
Peach, canned in natural juice	30	Papaya	60		
Apples	34	Figs	61		
Pears	41	Pineapple	66		
Dried Apricots	32				
Grapes	43				
Coconut	45				
Coconut Milk	41				
Kiwi Fruit	47				
Oranges	40				
Strawberries	40				
Prunes	29				

Dairy

Low GI		Medium GI		High GI	
Whole milk	31	Icecream	62		
Skimmed milk	32				
Chocolate milk	42				
Sweetened yoghurt	33				
Artificially Sweetened Yoghurt	23				
Custard	35				
Soy Milk	44				

Below are a few good websites which you can visit to learn more about the Glycemic Index.

http://www.glycemicindex.com/

http://www.southbeach-diet-plan.com/glycemicfoodchart.htm

http://www.health.harvard.edu/newsweek/Glycemic_index_and_glycemic_load_for_100_foods.htm

http://www.weightlossresources.co.uk/diet/gi_diet/glycaemic_index_tables.htm

http://lowcarbdiets.about.com/od/whattoeat/a/glycemicindlist.htm

Bibliography

1.   Natural Approach to Diabetes. Dr. Sarah Brewer, 2005. Piatkus Books Ltd.

2.   Encyclopedia of Natural Medicine Revised 2nd Edition: Michael Murray N.D. and Joseph Pizzorno N.D.

3.   Alternative Medicine: The Definitive Guide; Second Edition: Larry Trivieri, JR Editor, Introduced by Burton Goldberg.

4.   Alternative Cures: Bill Gottlieb

5.   Kilham C 2012. Does America Have a Diabetes Death Wish? Online Article.

6.   Shaw G 2012. How to Avoid – and even reverse – diabetes. Online Article.

7.   Newscore 2012. What's the Difference Between Type 1 and Type 2 Diabetes? Online Article

More Books by John McArthur

Hypothyroidism
Hypothyroidism: The Hypothyroidism Solution. Hypothyroidism Natural Treatment and Hypothyroidism Diet for Under Active Or Slow Thyroid, Causing Weight Loss Problems, Fatigue, Cardiovascular Disease. John McArthur (Author), Cheri Merz (Editor)

Fibromyalgia And Chronic Fatigue
Fibromyalgia And Chronic Fatigue: A Step-By-Step Guide For Fibromyalgia Treatment And Chronic Fatigue Syndrome Treatment. Includes Fibromyalgia Diet And Chronic Fatigue Diet And Lifestyle Guidelines. John McArthur (Author), Cheri Merz (Editor)

Yeast Infection
Candida Albicans: Yeast Infection Treatment. Treat Yeast Infections With This Home Remedy. The Yeast Infection Cure. John McArthur (Author)

Heart Disease
Hypertension - High Blood Pressure: How To Lower Blood Pressure Permanently In 8 Weeks Or Less, The Hypertension Treatment, Diet and Solution. John McArthur (Author)

Cholesterol Myth: Lower Cholesterol Won't Stop Heart Disease.

Healthy Cholesterol Will. Cholesterol Recipe Book & Cholesterol Diet. Lower Cholesterol Naturally Keep Cholesterol Healthy. John McArthur (Author), Cheri Merz (Editor)

Heart Disease Prevention and Reversal: How To Prevent, Cure and Reverse Heart Disease Naturally For A Healthy Heart. John McArthur (Author)

Diabetes

Diabetes Diet: Diabetes Management Options. Includes a Diabetes Diet Plan with Diabetic Meals and Natural Diabetes Food, Herbs and Supplements for Total Diabetes Control. Delicious Recipes. John McArthur (Author), Corinne Watson (Editor)

Diabetes Cooking: 93 Diabetes Recipes for Breakfast, Lunch, Dinner, Snacks and Smoothies. A Guide to Diabetes Foods to Help You Prepare Healthy Delicious ... Diabetic Meals and Natural Diabetes Food) John McArthur (Author), Corinne Watson (Editor)

Stress and Anxiety

From Stressful to Successful in 4 Easy Steps: Stress at Work? Stress in Relationship? Be Stress Free. End Stress and Anxiety. Excellent Stress Management, Stress Control and Stress Relief Techniques. John McArthur (Author)

Anxiety and Panic Attacks: Anxiety Management. Anxiety Relief.

The Natural And Drug Free Relief For Anxiety Attacks, Panic Attacks And Panic Disorder. John McArthur (Author), Cheri Merz (Editor)

Back and Neck Pain
The 15 Minute Back Pain and Neck Pain Management Program: Back Pain and Neck Pain Treatment and Relief 15 Minutes a Day No Surgery No Drugs. Effective, Quick and Lasting Back and Neck Pain Relief. John McArthur (Author)

Arthritis
Arthritis: Arthritis Relief for Osteoarthritis, Rheumatoid Arthritis, Gout, Psoriatic Arthritis, and Juvenile Arthritis. Follow The Arthritis Diet, Cure and Treatment Free Yourself From The Pain. John McArthur (Author)

Depression
How to Break the Grip of Depression: Read How Robert Declared War On Depression ... And Beat It! John McArthur (Author)

Pregnancy
Pregnancy Nutrition: Pregnancy Food. Pregnancy Recipes. Healthy Pregnancy Diet. Pregnancy Health. Pregnancy Eating and Recipes. Nutritional Tips and 63 Delicious Recipes for Moms-to-Be. Corinne Watson (Author), John McArthur (Author)

Pregnancy and Childbirth: Expecting a Baby. Pregnancy Guide. Pregnancy What to Expect. Pregnancy Health. Pregnancy Eating and Recipes. Cheri Merz (Author), John McArthur (Author)

Allergies

Allergy Free: Fast Effective Drug-free Relief for Allergies. Allergy Diet. Allergy Treatments. Allergy Remedies. Natural Allergy Relief. John McArthur (Author), Cheri Merz (Editor)